PHYSICIANS HEALED

Personal, inspiring and compelling
stories of fifteen courageous physicians
who do not prescribe contraception

Edited by Cleta Hartman

One More Soul
1846 North Main Street
Dayton, Ohio 45405-3832

(937) 279-5433
(800) 307-7685

OMSoul@OMSoul.com
www.OMSoul.com

© 1998 One More Soul. All rights reserved.
ISBN: 0-9669777-0-X

CONTENTS

FOREWORD

Scores of volumes have been written and speeches delivered concerning the Church's longstanding doctrine regarding pro-creation. (Pope John Paul II has certainly been at the forefront of those seeking to announce and explain this teaching.)

Perhaps the most persuasive of all arguments in support of the Church's teaching is the stellar example of those who <u>are</u> being faithful to the mandate of Christ. Married couples do incalculable good by living and spreading far and wide the "good news" of the Church's doctrine.

Take those couples, align them with members of the clergy and the medical profession who spare no effort in sharing the inherent beauty of Jesus' command as imparted and guarded by His Church, and witness the result: inspiring fidelity to the teaching of the Catholic Church which in turn calls others to look afresh at just what the Church expects and requires of her children — and what God expects and requires of <u>all</u> peoples. These clergy and health care professionals follow the lead of married couples and help to reinforce in their own specific ways the truth revealed by God which these spouses live out day to day.

You will note in reading these edifying personal "stories" two distinct, but related facts. First, <u>it is possible</u> to accept and live by the Church's teachings pertaining to the transmission of human life. Yes, those who do may be openly scorned for holding fast to the revealed truth of the Church's doctrine. Yet, it is possible not only to remain steadfast in the truth, but also to be a willing mouthpiece for the Holy Spirit as He uses those who are receptive to pass along the saving and enriching message found in *Humanae Vitae*.

Second, <u>there is the opportunity for conversion</u>. Never must it be said that those who promote and defend *Humanae Vitae* have "written off" as hopeless someone who currently advocates the contraceptive mentality. Those physicians whose accounts are captured in this work could have easily been considered "lost." But, thanks to God's grace, the prayers and sacrifices of many and their own searching for the truth, these physicians eventually yielded to the enduring wisdom of the Church.

Father Charles M. Mangan
Diocese of Sioux Falls

INTRODUCTION

"This day I call heaven and earth as witnesses against you that I have set before you life and death, blessings and curses. Now choose life, so that you and your children may live." (Deut 30:19)

A couple of years ago, on a long airplane ride from Colorado Springs to Orlando, my husband John, a family physician, was faced with a similar situation. There was a clear choice with profound consequences before him — a choice between continuing to prescribe contraceptives or refusing to do so. As he struggled with his decision, I was gripped with fear. I feared the financial consequences and the emotional cost this decision would surely bring to our lives. Could John be happy with a practice made up of only children and the aged? Will we have to sell our new house? What in the world would his partners say about this? So many scary thoughts terrorized my mind and made my heart sink — all along knowing that **once John formed the question clearly in his mind, there could only be one answer: he would stop prescribing contraceptives**.

None of the dire consequences I imagined came true. John continues to see many patients in their years of fertility, and he enjoys this part of his practice even more than ever. We were not forced into bankruptcy; our income experienced no change at all. His Christian partners may have been puzzled by John's decision not to prescribe contraceptives, but they were tolerant of him. To the casual observer, nothing much had changed in our lives. But to John and me, everything was changed.

The decision has brought peace to John and a renewal in his enthusiasm for the practice of medicine and even in our relationship with each other and with our children. Everywhere we look — newspapers, scripture readings, nature — confirms the righteousness of John's decision, and we never looked back except in gratitude that we had been given a second chance to live our lives in a way which would be pleasing to God. **It became a defining moment in our life.**

Yet we felt very alone in our stand against the culture of our world. Our friends blindly stood by us, but they did not understand. John's partners — all strong Christians — although supporting John's right to change the way he practiced medicine, were skeptical about whether the changes were necessary or even good for his patients. Even members of our church seemed to distance themselves from us, perhaps fearing we might introduce the subject of contraception into casual conversation.

Feeling rather marginalized but also feeling the attraction of radically affecting our culture, John and I traveled to the Pope Paul VI Institute in Omaha, Nebraska, to learn more about Natural Family Planning. As he learned how he, as a Medical Consultant, could provide support to couples using Natural Family Planning, and I learned how to teach the Ovulation Method of NFP to interested couples, a wonderful thing happened. Between hours of lectures and studying, **we became aware that we were encircled by new friends,** all having undergone the same transformation we had recently experienced and also fully understanding the ramifications this change had brought to our lives. Relaxing between lectures, we entertained each other with "our stories" of journeys toward not prescribing contraceptives. Listening to their stories, **I was struck by several things: the great impact even one person's witness can have on another's moral decisions, the tremendous power of the clergy to influence the faithful, the isolation of many physicians and, finally, the secure peace that derives from good and wise decisions.**

John and I carried our friends' stories in our minds and hearts as we returned home to Kissimmee. **Their stories**

were both our encouragement and our challenge, bringing us comfort and directing our future. We know we have become better people for having heard them — recounted painfully, honestly, informally over coffee and pie.

Fifteen of these stories have been gathered and published here in the hope that other physicians will be strengthened in their stand against the use of contraceptives. The physicians, who generously gave of their non-existent "free" time to write their personal stories, courageously opened their past lives and decisions to scrutiny and possible criticism. It was done freely, as a gift to their fellow physicians, to encourage and reassure them that many others have successfully made this journey, and that they wish them well.

If "many are called, but few are chosen," then the following fifteen physicians are truly the chosen few. I am so grateful to these men and women for wholeheartedly answering my plea to tell their stories, for revisiting the many painful decisions that accompanied their journeys, and lastly, for allowing their lives to be openly revealed on paper. Their journeys have inspired me and I will be forever in their debt.

I am grateful also to Steve Koob, the Director of One More Soul, for publishing this collection of stories. With persistence and patience, he prodded, encouraged, corrected and directed me on more than a few occasions. And Steve has done it with style and grace. I thank him for giving me this forum, which has been a journey of faith for me as well.

For the honor and glory of God, the Father, the Son, and the Holy Spirit.

Cleta Hartman

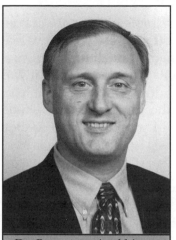

Dr. Baggot received his medical degree from the University of Illinois in 1982, and completed a residency in OB/GYN and Maternal Fetal Medicine and Human Genetics.

Dr. Baggot is on staff at the Pope Paul VI Institute in Omaha, Nebraska where he has a special interest in preventing birth defects and miscarriage with pre-conception care.

Paddy Jim is single. He says his wife is TBA (to be announced!)

MEA CULPA, MEA CULPA, MEA MAXIMA CULPA*

Paddy Jim Baggot MD

I decided to go into OB/GYN in 1988. I spoke with my god-father before I interviewed for the program and he suggested that I should tell the chairman before he hired me that I would not do abortions. And so when the chairman offered me the job, I told him that we have to understand that I would not do abortions. He said, "Will you take care of the complications?" I said, "I have no problem with that." He said, "Fine." He hired me.

What I didn't realize at the time was that he was a strong proponent of abortion and felt very strongly about them. He had fired nurses for refusing to participate in abortions and he had reportedly hounded previous residents out of the program for not participating in abortions. People could be fired for no reason from this residency program. Initially, I was the only one who did not do abortions. By the time I finished the program, about two-thirds of the residents didn't do abortions.

The fact that Catholic medical schools participate in contraception sets an example that is widely noticed. I knew that many Catholic residencies performed sterilizations and prescribed birth control pills. The rationalization was that it was "training." So I decided that I could do contraception, at least while I was in training. I felt from the beginning that when I was done with my training, I would probably have to stop prescribing birth control pills because I would no longer have the "training" excuse.

During my residency I read a lot of books, as I always do. I read all the major textbooks of obstetrics and gynecology and a lot of manuals as well. As I read more and more, my views on contraception started to change. I first began to realize that the IUD was an abortifacient. I might have put in one IUD, or maybe two, but after that I didn't put in any more. *Mea culpa.*

About halfway through my residency, the Norplant came out on the market and there was a tremendous hullabaloo about this. It was like the appearance of Windows 95. My GYN endocrinology professor told me that the progestin in the Norplant would suppress ovulation. I probably put in one or two, but then I started to have some doubts about whether this was a contraceptive or was it really an abortifacient. I was reading and hearing about patients who were having a lot of bleeding problems; the Norplant was notorious for bleeding problems. What really piqued my interest was the point that some women bleed every month with Norplant. It dawned on me that if they are bleeding every month, then they are ovulating. If they are ovulating, then the mechanism may be abortifacient. *Mea culpa.*

I started to believe that some of what was in the GYN textbooks, and some of what my teachers were telling, was not accurate from a pro-life perspective. At times it seemed more like propaganda from Planned Parenthood. One professor told me that termination of embryonic life before a gestational age of four weeks was not really an abortion because a placenta had not yet formed. A current example is literature about "post-coital" or "emergency contraception." Two recent issues of the New England Journal carried promotional pieces on emergency contraception as a way to "prevent" an unwanted pregnancy. These incidents seem to indicate that scientific accuracy, and even honest counseling of patients, may at times be sacrificed.

During our residency we had a rape protocol which included "post-coital contraception." Unfortunately, I must confess I did not have the intestinal fortitude to oppose it. *Mea culpa.*

Toward the end of my residency, I began to question whether oral contraceptive pills were not, in fact, abortifacient. Reviewing what I knew about contraceptives, and how I had been deceived about the abortifacient nature of other "contraceptives," the conclusion seemed inescapable that they were indeed abortifacient. Luckily, only months remained in my residency. In six months all the prescriptions I had written would run out and I would no longer be responsible for chemical abortions. *Mea maxima culpa.*

In my residency we had a contraception clinic. Mothers would bring in their 14- year-old daughters and demand that they be put on the "Pill." How unfortunate for these girls that their mothers wouldn't dream of expecting chastity. How unfortunate that we chemically spayed them like rabbits when they were barely old enough to know what was going on. Some were quite naïve about sex. During my residency I began to question my rationale for contraception. I am still single, but I hope to marry after I find a wife. How pathetic it would be for my daughters if they knew I prescribed contraceptives. If contraceptives were unacceptable for my wife or daughters, then how could they be acceptable for my patients?

Now that I work at the Pope Paul VI Institute, most of the patients that I see use natural family planning rather than contraception. One of the most interesting and striking differences in this population is that the men seem to be much more supportive of their wives, and husbands come to many of the prenatal visits. I was shocked at this because before I came to Omaha I had never seen a husband come to a prenatal visit. In the ghetto area where I did my residency, many women came in to labor with their mother, or their sister, or their daughter or their girlfriend, but very few were attended by their husband. Some boyfriends would show up just at the time of delivery. With the birth of the child their manly faculties were demonstrated to their cronies. They could then immediately vanish. With Natural Family Planning this cavalier attitude is often replaced by total support on the part of the husbands.

In my residency we saw a lot of pre-cancerous disease of the cervix. This was attributed to multiple sex partners and early age of first intercourse. I am now aware of literature that suggests that the birth control pill itself, and not merely accompanying sexual practices, promotes development of pre-malignant cervical disease. Now that I work in an NFP-only OB practice, a serious cervical dysplasia is very rare.

I now realize that contraception is neither good nor necessary. May the Lord forgive me for those human embryos I eliminated with IUDs. Mea culpa. May the Lord forgive me for those human embryos I eliminated with Norplant. Mea culpa. May the Lord forgive me for those human embryos I eliminated with the rape protocol. Mea culpa. May the Lord forgive me for those human embryos I eliminated with birth control pills. *Mea maxima culpa.*

As physicians, we should realize that the Popes have far more wisdom on ethical issues than we could imagine. We can only appreciate their wisdom by following their teachings. We are not smart enough to overrule their infallible reasons. Eight years of medical training does not counterbalance 2000 years of Catholic tradition. To learn, we must adopt an open-minded attitude of humility and obedience.

Mea culpa, mea culpa, mea maxima culpa — Latin phrase meaning "through my fault, through my fault, through my most grievous fault" which signifies a formal acknowledgment of personal fault or error.

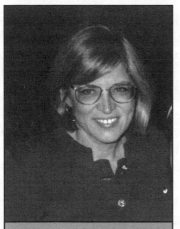

NEVER TOO LATE

Mary L. Davenport, MD

Dr. Mary Davenport, a Fellow of the American College of Obstetrics and Gynecology, graduated from Tufts Medical School in 1975 and completed her residency in Obstetrics and Gynecology at U.C. San Diego. She is now in a solo OB/GYN practice and maintains offices in Oakland and El Sobrante, California. Mary, a member of the Eastern Orthodox Church, and her husband Thomas Lifson have a ten-year-old son, Matthew.

My commitment to becoming an NFP-only medical practitioner cannot be easily separated from other aspects of my personal and spiritual life. When I entered my OB/GYN residency at U.C. San Diego in 1976, I never would have imagined that twenty years in the future I would not be prescribing contraception, and that I would have fully embraced natural family planning as a lifestyle for myself and my patients.

I grew up in Minneapolis, Minnesota, in the 1950s and 1960s as a daughter of a physician. From a young age I aspired to be a physician myself. My life was shattered at the age of eight when my father died of a heart attack. I had a child's faith in God and Jesus prior to this event, but after my father's death I became an atheist. I could not imagine how a good and loving God could take away my father. Although I went to a Congregational church while I was in my mother's household, it was because I was forced to, and I became cynical, hardened, and hypercritical of many aspects of Christianity. Nonetheless, despite my worldview, the habit of weekly churchgoing, participation in a church choir, and exposure to other Christians benefited me, although I definitely was not aware of this at the time. I was not exposed in this church, however, to a solid view of the Gospel and Scripture that would have been a real alternative to my belief system.

During my adolescence I was an aspiring intellectual. I found my life in Minnesota unbelievably boring and could not wait to go East to college. I developed an interest in Freudian psychology; my first introduction was at a Unitarian church to which my mother occasionally allowed me to go because I enjoyed the stimulating intellectual atmosphere and higher level of culture than my neighborhood church. I also found Kinsey's book on human sexuality at a home of a psychologist for which I was babysitting. Both were unbelievable spiritual poisons for a rebellious, ungrounded, unhappy young woman. I also discovered the power of sexuality at this time, and adopted a belief in sexual freedom as an ideology. No matter that underneath I was lonely and hurting, especially following the death of my mother at the age of seventeen; I thought I knew that sexual repression was unhealthy even though this worldview totally contradicted my own personal experience for the next twenty years.

I was at Smith College in the late sixties, a time of maximal social upheaval. I bounced around in my studies, but finally began taking premedical courses late in my college career. At this time I started using oral contraceptives for prevention of pregnancy, a practice I continued without interruption for the next twenty years, from the age of seventeen to thirty-seven. Throughout those twenty years, I also was chronically depressed, at times severely. I never correlated depression with the pill, and never would have even considered going off at the time, because of my certainty that I needed to avoid pregnancy, finish my education, and pursue my career.

Following graduation from Smith, I completed the necessary pre-med courses and volunteered in Boston at a newly opened abortion counseling center. Prior to the Roe v. Wade Supreme Court decision, this center shipped women to New York for abortions following New York's passage of its liberal state abortion law in 1970. There, I learned the pro-abortion lingo from the other well-meaning counselors- "It's just a blob of tissue," etc. I even paid a visit to one of America's first abortion centers, run by Dr. Bernard Nathanson. He aptly describes this place as "nightmarish" in his book, *The Hand of God*. I suppressed my feelings about this excursion, and adopted the extreme tolerance, even approval, of abortion that prevails in the medical profession. On applications for medical school, my essay on "Why I Want to Be a Doctor" was explicitly about wanting to make contraception and abortion available to women, and in the immediate pre-Roe v. Wade climate on the east coast, this was viewed by many in medicine as a good thing. I succeeded in obtaining admission to several medical schools, and chose Tufts in Boston.

Medical school went fairly well for me, and I was never personally exposed to abortion during this time. Following graduation from Tufts in 1975, I had a fairly good year in a rotating internship at Virginia Mason Hospital in Seattle, followed by residency in OB/GYN at U.C. San Diego. My live-in "boyfriend" was also a medical student with me, and we "matched" together in the internship and residency selection process (pretending we were engaged, although one probably doesn't need to do that anymore in the 1990s), pursuing our medical careers simultaneously in Massachusetts, Washington, and California. Taking oral contraceptives, as well as my values and priorities at the time, allowed me to prolong an essentially adolescent life-style well into my thirties.

At. U.C. San Diego, we did obstetrics during our internship year, and did not encounter abortion directly for yet another year. University Hospital had a top neonatal intensive care unit, and I did a research project on survival and gestational age, which at that time in 1976-77 were about 25% at 26 weeks. We were in a referral hospital, and worked valiantly to save the pregnancies of high-risk women, many delivering two or three months before their due date. U.C. San Diego was also a referral hospital for late abortions, and women were sent here from all over the Southwest. The prevailing technique at the time was direct saline and prostaglandin injection into the uterus, and in my second year of residency we would "see one, do one, teach one" as with all medical techniques that we learned. Ultrasound was new and fairly primitive at the time, but useful in the absence of good pregnancy dating; however, it could be off by two to even four weeks. We were supposed to turn away pregnant women who were over twenty-four weeks, which was felt to be approximately the lower limit of viability and also the limit of California law as it was interpreted at that time.

Along with my fellow residents and my "theoretical" approval of abortion and desire to help women with unwanted pregnancies, I learned how to inject saline and prostaglandin. Of course we had no exposure to medical ethics, no discussion about whether this procedure was right or wrong, and no discussion whatsoever that generations of physicians for almost 2000 years had taken an oath to ostracize any physician who performed this procedure, and that it was explicitly illegal from the founding of this republic until just five years prior. This crossing over a line, the taking of human life in medical practice, was reduced to the level of a "technique."

As junior residents, we were expected to help deliver the dead fetuses. This took place on the gynecology floor in the patient's hospital bed. It was fairly gruesome, with heads of dead babies getting stuck in the patient's cervixes, retained placentas, and lots of blood. On one memorable evening a young woman who measured more than thirty centimeters (consistent with a more than thirty-week pregnancy) had been injected by one of my young colleagues without an ultrasound by the explicit orders of one of the faculty physicians. The two of us involved in the delivery were most distressed to see a perfectly formed dead thirty-three week baby, with lanugo hair, unfused eyelids, and numerous post-viability features — more mature than the "pre-viable" dead fetuses that we forced ourselves to tolerate. Now this was a baby for whom we might be performing a Cesarean section to save! I helped initiate a protest among the residents, and we residents did not do any more abortion injections while I was in training, but continued to help deliver the dead babies aborted by faculty members. The faculty member involved spoke of this event as a "tragedy," but in retrospect it was most likely to appease our slightly more tender sensibilities. It would not be long before abortions right through the ninth month for "health" would be available to virtually anyone in California in some facilities with no monitoring or oversight from public health authorities.

I performed a few first-trimester abortions as a senior resident, but most abortions of this type were not done in teaching hospitals. Although not as deeply disturbing at a gut level as mid-trimester abortions, I felt vaguely uneasy during this clinical experience. Good medical procedure demanded that we inspect the "products of conception" that we had suctioned out of the uterus, to count the limbs and head and make sure the evacuation was complete. I had first seen this done at Nathanson's clinic in New York. I found this practice revolting. Why couldn't we just let it go into the specimen bag and leave it at that? I began to realize what a pathological effect that doing abortions, as well as my self-image as an abortionist, was having on me when I ran into a friend from medical school years. She asked, "Do you have babies?" and I blurted out, "No, I kill babies," and we were both equally shocked at this exchange. I had a friend who was a Zen Buddhist, and read a book by his spiritual teacher, Roshi Philip Kapleau, *To Cherish All Life*. Although it made a stronger case for vegetarianism than against abortion, it did address the seriousness of taking human life. I began a ten-year habit of searching for the meaning of life by travel in Asia and the study and practice of eastern religions.

Following completion of my residency, I moved to Portland, Oregon, with my "boyfriend" where I went to work for the Kaiser Hospital system and he went into private practice. At Kaiser at this time, one third of the pregnancies ended in abortion. When women had a positive pregnancy test, they were asked by the receptionist, "Do you want to continue or terminate?" and were referred to the appropriate clinic. I performed perhaps one hundred or two hundred first trimester abortions while I was at Kaiser, in morning-long clinics, doing five to ten at a time once a month, as well as occasional clinics of mid-trimester abortions done by digoxin intrauterine injection, prostaglandin suppository, and vaginal delivery. I did not connect my worsening depression with doing abortions, although it was definitely a factor.

Now that I was done with my residency, I needed to face the fact that my partner and I were definitely out of "love." Whatever feelings I might have had were killed off by years of sterilized sex on the pill (Even the Kinsey Institute — the premier sex research facility — recently put out a paper on how a large percentage of women on the pill lose their sexual desire.), and lack of normal progression of this relationship to marriage and children. The hope that finishing my medical residency and improvement in material circumstances would make me feel better was not realistic.

I began to seek out help for my depression beyond conventional psychotherapy, and traveled to Esalen, the well-known alternative psychology center in Big Sur, California, in 1982. It was there that I encountered some tapes of Mother Teresa, who gave a very clear testimony on abortion being murder at something called the "International Conference on Transpersonal Psychology" in Bombay, and these teachings reached me at Esalen! I made a decision at that time to perform no more abortions. After more exposure to what were essentially eastern religious teachings, I decided to leave Kaiser, Oregon, and my partner of ten years, and move to Berkeley, which was a new age center. My poisonous self-absorption persisted. I lectured on "embodiment" and pre- and perinatal psychology (birth and prenatal memories) in Europe and the U.S., traveled to the USSR to meet with people delivering new age "superbabies" with various occultic prenatal and birth techniques, as well as developing an interest in natural birth. In spite of my vow to not do abortions, I ended up performing them in order to get a job as an OB/GYN physician at a county hospital. I was persuaded that "if I didn't do them, somebody else would." This felt terrible, and I finally notified my colleagues that as of January 1, 1984, I would do no more.

I was in my late thirties when I quit the pill and noted an immediate improvement in my mood and energy level. Quitting the pill also unleashed normal female hormones, and I began to experience the desire to be pregnant, something that had been entirely absent in the past. I cannot blame all of my former psychopathology on the pill, but it definitely contributed to many of my unhealthy tendencies. Soon after this, an old high school friend, Thomas Lifson, came back into my life, we fell in love and married, and we had our son Matthew in 1988.

I had gone into private practice in 1985, and ended up being in solo practice to separate myself physically and financially from the performance of abortions. This was not so easy in the Bay area, where most OB/GYNs perform abortions, unlike many other parts of the United States. My practice attracted a number of devout evangelical Christians who sought natural birth, and a physician who didn't perform abortions. These patients, who home-schooled their children, and had large families, were the first people I met who didn't use contraception. I was completely fascinated with these Christians, although initially I couldn't imagine living like that! I also was growing discontented with my new age belief system, and discovered when I gave my "embodiment" talk in 1989, integrating Eastern religions and pre- and perinatal psychology, I didn't actually believe what I was saying any more. I decided at that moment not to give any more talks that I knew weren't the truth. Giving birth to my son put me in touch with the fact that he was perfectly designed, not by an impersonal "force," but by a loving Creator. I experienced becoming a mother as a wonderful blessing, of which I was totally undeserving and unworthy, but privileged to experience.

I started inhabiting Christian book stores, and came across the journal of the Spiritual Counterfeits Project, a Berkeley organization dedicated to evangelizing persons like myself who were believers in new age and Eastern religions. I came across a chart outlining the differences between the "New Age Worldview" and "Biblical Worldview." Having a young child made me hyper-aware of dangers in the world. I had just heard a lecture on satanic ritual abuse, something that I had not even known existed. Prior to my son's birth, I had been lulled into believing that there was no such a thing as evil, but good and evil were like dark and light, different aspects of the same reality. But my "Biblical Worldview" chart said that there was such a thing as sin, which was disobedience and falling away from the will of God. At that moment, everything clicked into place for me, and I saw myself as desperately in need of a Savior.

I called the hot line with the Spiritual Counterfeits Project, and began going to a Conservative Baptist Church with a wonderful pastor and mentor, Bill Kellog, much to the horror of my friends and colleagues. I began to get an appreciation for the Word of God, something for which I will forever be grateful. My husband was teaching in Japan for several months at the time, and I was able to spend quite a bit of time in Bible study and going to church at this time without creating family conflict. Also, my son, although just three years old, became a believer in Jesus at this time.

It took me some time after my becoming Christian to experience contraception as an issue. It was not a real issue at that time in evangelical Christian circles. Although some Christian physician organizations have oaths stating that they believe that life begins at conception, the vast majority of Christian physicians in primary care and gynecology prescribe hormonal contraception, which at times prevents implantation of the embryo. I never really questioned this fact, which I learned in my residency. I continued to insert IUDs also, seizing upon newer data that indicate that the copper IUDs work as true contraceptives at least some of the time. I toyed with the idea that the beginning of life really had to be implantation, for the mother's role was critical, and the circumstances of twinning and blighted ova support this view. I also became more active in pro-life activities, debating pro-abortion people in front of Berkeley premedical students with Gregg Cunningham of the Center for Bioethical Reform, who later challenged me on my prescribing the pill. My initial reaction was anger and annoyance at his persistence — and his logic.

I became a board member for AAPLOG, an organization of pro-life OB/GYNs. During the first few years of my membership oral contraception was not discussed, because it is a totally divisive issue among pro-life physicians of various stripes. When I joined, I asked if one could prescribe IUDs, oral contraceptives, and post-coital contraception and be a member of the organization. I was told the organization existed to fight surgical and medical abortion of established pregnancies, and that the IUDs and hormonal contraction didn't violate that principal. Like the Christian medical groups I belonged to, AAPLOG used the same terminology about protecting life after conception in its pledge. This didn't make sense to me, but I figured if the distinguished physicians who started this organization at the time of Roe v. Wade could live with that contradiction, I could too. I later found out that many AAPLOG doctors actually do not believe that oral contraceptives act as abortifacients, which was a complete surprise to me!

In 1995, I joined with two partners to form Grace Medical Group, an explicitly Christian practice. At the time, we became aware of referring for abortions as a moral issue, and stopped doing this. As a consequence the two of us who were OB/GYNs were not awarded a large contract to perform obstetrical services for a nearby community hospital because we wouldn't have a "reciprocal" relationship with Planned Parenthood and refer abortions to them. The family practice physician who worked with us had made a decision to not give contraceptives to unmarried women. This decision had created tensions for him in his job at a Christian clinic in Mississippi, but was not a problem for our practice because the two of us who were OB/GYNs would prescribe contraception for anyone! My other partner, an OB/GYN, would not prescribe post-coital contraception. I did not see much difference between oral contraceptives used in the normal and post-coital fashion. We thought at the time that we were about as pro-life as any physicians in the Bay area could realistically be.

However, I began to encounter more people within the pro-life movement who did not use contraception. Their families seemed to exude a special love and grace. I read more deeply, and found that all Christians prior to 1930 regarded contraception as an evil. Kimberly Hahn's tapes on the scriptural and natural law arguments against contraception were very persuasive to me. Around this time I encountered my very first OB/GYN physicians who did not prescribe contraception in their medical practice — Dr. Carolina Braga and Dr. Murphy Goodwin. Although they were not generalist OB/GYNs in private practice like myself, I was amazed. I could not imagine putting this into effect in my own medical practice despite my attraction to this point of view.

Although the Conservative Baptist Church had provided a wonderful exposure to Scripture, I did not feel totally comfortable there and began to study other types of Christianity and other types of worship. For awhile I attended an Evangelical Covenant Church, and was very interested in the charismatic movement and healing. I also felt a deep attraction toward Catholicism because of the pro-life movement and because I believed in the Real Presence of Christ in the Eucharist and longed to experience this. I began to pray that God lead me to the right church.

During the summer of 1995, while attending a summer family bible camp, I wandered into a place in the Santa Cruz Mountains called the Conciliar Press Bookstore. I had initially thought it was a Catholic bookstore, but it turned out to be an Orthodox bookstore, run by a wonderful group of people who had formerly been a Protestant congregation. I spent the first of many small fortunes on books from this store, and found a wealth of material I had never previously encountered on the Fathers of the Church, saints and martyrs, as well as the story of this group's spiritual journey. I stayed up all night reading, and attended my first Divine Liturgy the next morning. That Thursday morning in August, there was a full choir and quite a few people at St. Peter and Paul's Church. The walls of the church were covered with icons. The psalms and music as they were sung were of a depth that I had never encountered before. I stood before the iconostasis and altar, in awe of such purity and holiness. I began weeping uncontrollably, and fell to the floor, deeply aware of my own sinfulness and aware as never before of God's presence and love. I believed this was the answer to my prayers, and joined the Orthodox Church shortly thereafter.

In 1996, I became exposed to contemporary natural family planning when I attended a California conference for NFP professionals. I learned for the first time — after twenty years in OB/GYN — that NFP was not the Rhythm method, and that it worked 98-99% of the time! Despite my board certification in OB/GYN and being a fellow in ACOG, I had never encountered Odeblad's voluminous work on cervical mucus. Here was a very important body of scientific knowledge to which I was not exposed for many years of medical practice, to my great regret and the detriment of my patients. I made contact with a wonderful group of Creighton-method NFP instructors based at St. Rose Hospital, which was only fifteen minutes away from my office in Oakland. Shortly thereafter I enthusiastically began instruction in NFP and began to use it myself. At this time I still could not imagine giving up prescribing contraception in my medical practice, even though I could see the many benefits of NFP. Dr. Joe Stanford, a speaker at the conference, encouraged me to go through the program at Pope Paul VI Institute in Omaha to learn more, even though I would have to go as an "auditor" because I didn't meet the ethical standards of not prescribing or referring for contraception to become an official NFP Medical Consultant.

It took me more than a year to get to Omaha. During that year, the burden of prescribing contraception weighed more heavily on me, especially facilitating the immoral lifestyle of unmarried women. Was I helping them waste their lives and desecrate their bodies? But then I would ask myself — wasn't that better than an unwanted pregnancy, illegitimacy, or possible abortion? This topic came up for me a lot in confession. I once told a priest that I felt like an old whore instructing younger ones. What a horrible legacy to pass on — infecting the next generation with the dissipated, baby-boomer lifestyle of the sexual revolution. This is something I would never want for my family or friends. Why was I doing it to my patients? The NFP instructors came to our office to offer classes to our patients. They would encourage me and showed me testimonies of physicians who had switched to NFP-only practices. I found these stories most exciting! Dr. José Férnàndez came to speak at St. Rose Hospital, and took me aside. "God's calling you to holiness," he said, and I started to cry and couldn't look at him. I had never heard another physician speak to me in that way before.

On arriving at the Pope Paul VI Institute, I met two other OB/GYNs who had NFP-only practices, one in a fully-Catholic setting and another in a mixed practice with other contracepting OB/GYNs, Dr. Anna-Marie Manning and Dr. Stephen Hickner. I asked how they worked out the mechanics of their practice, and became aware that I could do it too! They told me that the other physicians in my area would think I was crazy, but that was all right. I felt as if I had found soul mates. Also, Dr. Tom Hilgers, who was in charge of the Pope Paul VI program, said that to become a Medical Consultant, the switch to an NFP-only practice did not have to happen instantly. That relieved me because I was concerned about informing my patients properly, my relationship with them, and not abandoning them. I knew that I was going to have to make a decision, and set a date three months later, when all contraception and sterilization would be gone from my practice. I then sent a fax to my medical partner in Oakland from my motel in Omaha, prayed, and hoped she would understand.

The peace I have felt since becoming an NFP-only medical practitioner has been immeasurable. The difficulties along the way have thus far been relatively minor. I have become an evangelist for NFP, and will talk about it at length to anyone! I now am more sure that I am helping, not compromising, the women under my care. In exposing them to NFP, I can help them appreciate their power to give life, and to love and respect God.

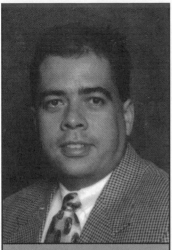

Dr. Fernández, currently on faculty at the St. Anthony Hospital Family Practice Residency Program in Oklahoma City, Oklahoma, graduated from the University of Florida College of Medicine in 1991. After completing a residency in Family Practice, Dr. Fernández worked with Mercy Hospital in Miami, Florida.

While living in Florida, Dr. Fernández was instrumental in reactivating the Florida Physician's Guild in many parts of the state and was honored to receive the Respect Life Award from the Archdiocese of Miami.

Jose and his wife Lucia are the parents of three young daughters, Olivia, Sofia and Natalia.

FAITH, HOPE AND LOVE
THE STEPPING STONES
OF MY LIFE

Jose R. Fernández, MD

One never knows where the winding road of life will take you. I certainly never thought that understanding human sexuality and the Catholic Church's role on this topic would impact my life as it has.

For me, growing up in a middle class immigrant family with strong family values and a Catholic upbringing, I thought I possessed all I needed for success and happiness. I, as so many other Catholics, thought that going to church on Sunday, confession when you really did something bad and participating in some church activities was all that one needed to be a "good" Catholic. I came to find out that I could not have been farther from the truth!

Back in the late 1980s, a good priest friend of mine showed me his rose garden, which was full of weeds, and he shared with me that we would not only remove the weeds from his garden, but also from the garden of my life. You see, that rose garden represented all the material things in my life. I possessed many things, everything that made me self-sufficient, especially all of my accomplishments, which filled me with great pride. These very things had become the weeds in the garden of my life.

Because of my self-sufficiency, I had no real need of God. And on the inside I was beginning to feel its effect as I experienced a sense of emptiness. This emptiness was brought about because the weeds in my life towered over the few rose petals left on the stem. Indeed, God now only played a distant role in directing my life journey, but worse off, I did not even know it! As the weeds tried to choke off the remnants of faith, hope and love I had instilled in me long ago, I was slowly led to the realization of who I would become once again. Fortunately, I had been planted in fertile ground—my faith; I had a Master Gardener—Our Lord; and I had the nourishment of life-giving water—the Holy Spirit. Now, as if the scales had been removed from my eyes, I began to see that in order for me to live and thrive I needed to surrender to the Master Gardener and allow the transformation of my life to take place.

So it was that on that day my priest friend was dutifully carrying out what he was ordained to do only a few years earlier. He simply was gathering another lost sheep into the fold. If only I would have had a glimpse as to the fullness of his message in this gentle parable of Life, and most importantly the deep impact those words would eventually have on my life. I had no real clue to its significance, as this was just prior to starting my medical education. Now, I can see how God's hands were ever so slowly pruning a new sensitivity, a new way of looking at life.

My first challenge occurred in my second year of medical school during an ethics class. I remember that no matter what was being discussed, there was never a right or wrong. My professors simply provided a way for us to substantiate whatever the individual or group thought was right or wrong, a sort of moral relativism. I was constantly reminded that one's bag of morals and life ethics should be left at the doorway to medical education, to possibly never be picked back up again.

Looking back at it now, I realize that there were many casualties during that phase of our educational system — the worst part was that most grew numb and never realized what they lost. For many, the "claims ticket" has never been drawn and today they wonder why they are so disenchanted with the medical profession. The numbness for many has never left!

A few years later, I found myself as a third year resident in a Family Practice Residency program just a few months from completing my residency program. I was regarded as competent and caring and was looking forward to a bright future. By this time I was married with two beautiful girls, attended Sunday Mass regularly and even taught Sunday school.

At the beginning of my marriage, my wife and I used contraceptives for family planning, but after our first child we decided to use a sympto-thermal method of natural family planning as our preferred method. This decision was not based on faith, but more on our concerns for the side effects of the "pill" and the fact that my wife never took it consistently anyway. Although we were now using a natural method of family planning, I was generally not involved, but went along with it because I wanted to support my wife. For me, the days of abstinence were very difficult and frustrating — this would persist for many years.

I took this historical detour to point out the fact that I never thought my personal feelings about family planning would or should ever impact my practice of medicine. I was taught that I was there to serve my patients, whether they wanted a birth control pill or a tubal ligation. My personal feelings, and much less what my church taught on the subject, had nothing to do with the practice of medicine. And to be honest, I never knew what the Church really taught on this subject and, even if I knew it, I certainly thought that it would not or could not impact the way I practiced medicine.

So one day at the end of a rotation in the family practice residency program, one of my best friends asked me something that will forever be embedded in the roots of my being. "José, I know that you are a good doctor, but are you a Catholic doctor?". . . . This simple question threw me for a tailspin, but convicted me in a way I had never been convicted before in my life.

It took me a while to figure out what it meant, but from his stance on pro-life issues, I had a clue. In many ways I was back in the rose garden, one that was full of weeds now, but one in which I realized that a budding rose still lay there waiting to bloom.

I sought the counsel of many; most everyone I spoke with could not appreciate what the struggle was all about or why I wrestled with these issues, especially at this point in my life. I was made to feel that I would be abandoning my patients, I would be denying a service I always provided in the past. What would my patients say to me when I told them that I had stopped contracepting, and that I could no longer perform a vasectomy or a tubal ligation, just because my Church said so!

Of great encouragement to me were a first year resident and a senior faculty member in my residency program who were both convicted that there was only one way to practice medicine. Through it all, it was my wife that gave me the inner strength to know that I was on the right path. She was instrumental in helping me pick up the pieces, reassuring me that what I had decided was right, and in many ways showed me that I had not entered a profession called Medicine, but rather a vocation — a way of life. One which was very personal in which my values at home would and should impact my practice of medicine.

To my surprise, my patients did not feel abandoned. Some were curious as to why I had made this decision and some even admired me for standing up and believing in something. Yet, as a family physician, I felt incomplete. Obstetrics and Gynecology were an important part of the practice of Family Medicine which I enjoyed. Yet, no longer prescribing birth control pills or performing vasectomies limited my scope of practice. I felt incomplete.

About a year later, toward the end of my first year of teaching first-year medical students, I was keenly aware of something that had haunted me from my past. While teaching these students I felt that it was my responsibility to be a role model for each of them, and I was concerned about their future especially if they did not have the opportunity to learn that there was a right and wrong in medicine. I taught them that if they did not know where they stood on moral and ethical issues, their medical education would not be complete, so I began them on a course of exploration, one in which I was always sure to point out that there was a moral high ground. My boss at the time disagreed with me, and shared with me that my responsibility was simply to pass on information, nothing more. I also found, that working in a student health center in a major university, one could not provide gynecologic care if one did not prescribe birth control pills. So, my emptiness and incompleteness as a clinician grew. And so I moved on!

Now I was to start anew — in private practice. I was blessed to have a slow start in my practice which afforded me the time to do a lot of outside reading. I suppose this began my first attempts at restarting my Catholic formation where it had left off many years before. Since deciding to stop contracepting, my learning was simply an attempt to survive, but now I was much more systematic in my approach to understanding the Catholic faith. It was during this time that one of my best friends invited me to attend a course for physicians to become Medical Consultants for the Creighton Model of Natural Family Planning. Since I had the time and resources to do it, I was off to Omaha, Nebraska.

I never thought that in nine days I could both undergo a complete brain rinse and be made whole — as a man, father and physician. The time spent at the Pope Paul VI Institute was invaluable. I felt as if I was able to close one chapter of my life and began another. It was there that I truly learned what it meant to be pro-life and the difference between the culture of life and the culture of death. It was during this time that I realized what the contraceptive mentality was all about and how deeply it had affected me and my marriage.

Since that time I have become a strong advocate for natural family planning and the culture of life. I find myself each day trying to be more faithful to the God that loves me and forgives me continuously when I come to him. I have also come to realize that as a people, Catholics have been given tremendous graces through the sacraments — especially the Sacraments of Reconciliation and the Eucharist, and most importantly, the Sacrament of Marriage.

I realize that my best teacher on earth is my wife. She has taught me to be selfless, much in the same way my father has tried to live out his life. She has taught me to love, to give all that I possess, to be sensitive to the one we love and that lovemaking is multidimensional involving our spirituality, our bodies, our intellect, our words and our emotions. Through natural family planning we've come to understand our natural bodily rhythms. In using natural family planning, Our Lord had given us a method to use that enables us to recognize the times of fertility and infertility, while gently guiding us to work with Him to co-create. What a wonderful gift He has given us! This work has taught me that every child is a Blessing, as every one of our children has been to us. In conceiving our third child we were able to pray, communicate, and co-create with our Lord. We both understood how with complete knowledge of our fertility we could synchronize our bodies to the will of the Lord to fully appreciate His tremendous blessing from the very beginning of our child's life. . . WOW!

Once again I feel whole. I realize now that the rose garden of my life has fewer weeds, many more roses with full buds and some have bloomed. My profession has become a vocation — a way of life. Every day I am able to love a little more and forgive a little more. I have learned that there are certain things which cannot be compromised. For me, being a Catholic physician is all I know how to be, because my faith has pierced my heart and soul.

As one of the earliest Christian writings, the Didache, states: "There are two ways, one of life and one of death, and great is the difference between the two ways. The way of life is this: first, you shall love God, who created you; second, your neighbor as yourself. . . ." We must always choose the way of life, because if we do, then the Hand of God will be upon us. By choosing the way of life, our Lord will forever bless what we do in His name and many of life's most difficult decisions will become easy. How will you know this, you ask? Because when you choose Him and His will, you will feel His presence and peace in your life!

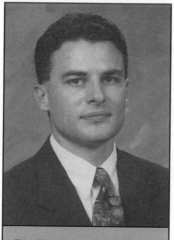

GETTING THROUGH RESIDENCY

Ron Ferris, MD

Dr. Ferris is currently a first year resident at the Via Christi Family Practice Residency in Wichita, Kansas. Twenty-seven years-old and a convert to Catholicism, he attended the University of Kansas School of Medicine, graduating in 1997. Ron and his wife Patricia are newlyweds.

I entered my residency training with the conviction that I would not prescribe oral contraceptives. This conviction came after my conversion to the Catholic Faith at the end of my senior year of college. I was attending Benedictine, a small Catholic college in northeast Kansas, and the reason I enrolled there was partially due to an interest to attend a small school.

I was blessed during college to be in a close group of friends who were faithful Catholics. They welcomed me even though I was pretty much a pagan being raised without any religion in my family. All five of the men in that group went on to seminary or religious life after college. I was very impressed by the witness of these five friends in their devotion to God and the truth that they lived by their faith. I understand now that it was only by the grace of God and their prayers, which I came to find out about later, that somehow began my conversion. The fishing net thrown by God brought them to their priestly vocations and me to be baptized a Catholic.

After becoming Catholic and graduating from college, I continued — with the help of friends — my formation in the faith. In medical school, I again was blessed with the friendship of a devout Catholic roommate who was literally contagious in his studying of the faith. As Scott Hahn (a well-known Catholic convert) says, "where you find a Catholic studying his faith, you will also find a Catholic that is contagious in their faith." I can definitely attest to that from experience in regard to my roommate. So, on top of our medical studies, we would "feed" each other different materials on various Church teachings, whatever we could get our hands on. A favorite of ours was John Paul II. With all of his encyclicals and a few of his books, he offered plenty of reading material to get us up to speed, so to speak.

I fortunately made it through medical school without getting tangled with too many snares of the devil regarding contraception, sterilization, and/or abortion. The clinic during our obstetrics/gynecology (OB/GYN) rotation was always a place where one had to be careful about getting drawn into participating with such an event, knowing the frequency of prescriptions written for contraception there. As a medical student, I saw two ways to evade this issue. The first way was to look at the day's schedule and plan to not participate with any patients coming in for contraceptives. The second option, if somehow the first was overlooked, was to plead ignorance and let the OB/GYN resident or attending take over. Medical students had limited experience filling out prescriptions at this point in our training anyway. The situation I wanted to avoid was where the medical student fills out the prescription and the resident or attending signs it. I did not want to actively cooperate in that situation.

As a medical student, I always felt some stress trying to avoid a possible bad confrontation with a resident or attending regarding my beliefs. One good piece of advice I received to prevent this ongoing stress of trying to avoid confrontations (which has not always been easy to live up to) is as follows: state your position clearly to the resident or attending the first time it arises, instead of letting the same stressful situation come up again and again. The outcome is usually better than you think and an ongoing burden is relieved.

Near the end of medical school, I decided to pursue a residency in Family Practice and now it was a matter of where. So I began interviewing.

I decided I would be up front about not prescribing the pill in my interviews for residency when I met specifically with the directors of the various programs. I asked myself "Did I really want to be part of a program if they could not accept me because of my religious beliefs?" This way, if any problems arose concerning the issue of contraception, I could simply state that I was in fact up front about it when I applied. I had a rehearsed line I would say to the residency director during interviews: "I'm an advocate of natural family planning and if I was accepted into the program, how do you think I would fit in?" For some of the interviews, it became obvious real quick by the puzzled look on his face that the program would be unprepared to handle somebody not prescribing and I would probably be regarded as a real whacko if I came there.

Match day came after much prayer and discernment from my fiancée and myself. Match day is the "big" day when all the fourth year medical students find out where they will be doing residency. It is all based on how we ranked different programs and how the programs ranked us. We matched at Via Christi Catholic Hospital in Wichita, Kansas — our first choice, a choice we felt directed by the Lord.

In order to head off any difficulties, I again met with the director of the residency, who already knew I would not prescribe contraception. He arranged it so that the front desk, responsible for scheduling patients, would not schedule anybody wanting hormonal contraceptives to see me. The arrangement has worked out fairly well. As time went on, the whole office staff, along with some of the other residents, has become aware of my position on contraception. An incident did happen early in the residency where a patient I was scheduled to see requested a Depo-Provera shot for contraception and my nurse administered it before I even saw the patient. (This was something done in the clinic with other residents and assumed to be fine in my case without any further discussion.) When I found out, I clarified my position with the nurse and he in turn related it to the other nursing staff, successfully preventing this situation from happening again.

A few times on my schedule, I have ended up getting a patient who failed to mention when she scheduled her appointment that she wanted birth control pills. These are always difficult situations for me. Normally, I would just have another resident take over, but one day a patient that I had already started to see couldn't be rescheduled to see another resident that day. That day in the end I had to explain the situation to the supervising faculty member, who took over and prescribed the contraceptive to the patient. Although I feared his reaction, the faculty member didn't really have much of a reaction towards the situation. However, I know having to take time from supervising a busy clinic and take care of my problem was obviously a burden. Not a good situation!

The patients in these situations usually indicate some understanding, but to what degree, it is unclear. They usually become quiet after I explain why I do not prescribe contraceptives and why I prefer using natural family planning methods. I tell them one of the reasons I do not prescribe is the abortifacient potential of all hormonal contraceptives; this probably is what leaves the patient wondering. I'm still working on the best way to present this kind of information along with NFP to the patient. My hope is that, with time, experience will help in this area.

I think it is a scandal — occurring on a widespread scale — to have family practice clinics, next to and associated with a Catholic hospital, distributing oral or other hormonal contraceptives. There are priests in our diocese that have become frustrated telling their parishioners that contraception is against the Catholic Church's teaching and for the parishioners to reply to the priest that they "got it from the Via Christi Family Practice Clinic."

I'm now halfway through my first year of residency and actually was able to get away recently to Omaha to become trained by the Pope Paul VI Institute. I received training both as a NFP Practitioner, which taught me how to teach NFP to couples, and as a NFP Medical Consultant, which taught me how to give technical medical support for couples using NFP and also be a physician referral source to support other NFP practitioners. The program was an immersion type of experience — and pretty much a boot camp — to become trained with the Creighton Model of NFP. I would highly recommend the consultant's program (for its in-depth training) to any physician. It has already helped me feel more secure while in formation toward being a NFP-only physician.

A couple of exciting events have happened since I returned from the program. I guess the word has been getting out that I was trained in NFP. I have had two of the first year residents talk with me, wanting to learn more about NFP. I couldn't believe it! It now looks like there are a good handful of residents (seven, including myself, in a program of 54 residents) that I know of whom are opposed to contraception. This is definitely encouraging and a start.

As an NFP practitioner, I am now training couples in the use of NFP. I am strengthened and sustained by this ministry. It gives me a sense of actively being part of the solution instead of part of the ever-increasing social problems in our society. I see the disintegration of the family happening all around us as one of many consequences of contraception that Pope Paul VI predicted in 1968 from his encyclical *Humanae Vitae*.

To anyone undertaking the fight against contraception and "fighting the good fight" as a physician, I pray that the Lord may sustain and strengthen you.

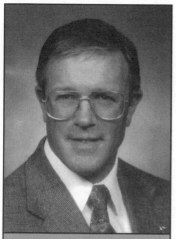

THE STONE WHICH THE BUILDERS REJECTED

John R. Hartman, MD

Dr. Hartman graduated from the University of Miami Medical School in 1976 and completed a residency in family medicine at Duke University in 1979. After serving three years in the U.S. Navy in Pensacola, Florida, he established a group family practice in Kissimmee, Florida in 1982.

Dr. Hartman is currently practicing with Heritage Family Physicians in Kissimmee where he joins with the other physicians of this group in authoring a column, entitled "Diary from a Week in Practice," which is a monthly feature in the journal of the "American Family Physician."

Dr. Hartman was named the Florida Family Physician of the Year in 1997 and was one of the ten finalists for the national honor the same year.

I have been Catholic all my life. Both my parents were Catholic and went to church each Sunday. This meant that, for my four siblings and me, we went to church on Sunday too — and we had better be well behaved about it. I went to Catholic schools for almost all of my elementary and high school years. I even was in a minor seminary for six years. So I guess you could say I was steeped in Catholicism.

In a sense I was, but in another sense, I wasn't. What I mean is, that when Pope Paul VI came out with his "infamous" encyclical *Humanae Vitae*, I was one of the many who were disappointed with the prohibition of the "pill," and one of the many who were confused about how he could have come to that conclusion. The "unitive and procre-

Married for 29 years, John and his wife Cleta are parents of three daughters, Karen, Heidi and Anne.

ative" meaning of sex was an abstract concept, of which I had little, if any, understanding. How much easier it would have been if the Pope had just followed the path of all the others, just read the "signs of the times" and endorsed contraception, content with putting some boundaries on its proper use.

Thus, it comes as no surprise that when my wife and I were to be married, and when the priest apologetically said that we didn't need to go into any great detail about the subject of family planning and contraception, I was just as happy to bypass this issue. The priest said all we needed to do was to submit the issue to our consciences and then he wouldn't need to spend any further time on it. I knew that I didn't want any hurdles placed in our path: our wedding was scheduled for Spring Break, just 4 $^1/_2$ weeks away, and there was no extra time in the schedule for special discussions. At the time, I knew we were making a shortcut and that it would be better to examine this in more depth, but the priest allowed us this short cut and we took it. Apparently we had just played into each other's hands! Sadly, I didn't discuss it further with my fiancée, or even consider how I could study more about the truth of that issue. I just did nothing. I allowed it to slip away from consciousness and was glad when it didn't keep cropping up to bother my conscience. (But deep inside I knew I had compromised myself and that I had just lied to myself about the truth of things.)

After that I didn't think much more about the contraception issue until my third year in medical school. (We had been married six years by then.) It was on the OB/GYN rotation that I was surprised and confronted. The issue was abortion. It was the practice of the hospital affiliated with the University of Miami to perform "terminations of pregnancies," or TOPs as they were called. As a third year medical student, I was expected to do a "history and physical" on a variety of patients admitted to the hospital, some of which were hospitalized for the purpose of abortion. I had feared this moment.

I was hoping once again to skirt the issue of abortion. While I was not outwardly distressed or saddened that others performed this killing, I knew I did not want to have that as part of my medical school experience. There began a struggle within me, and I could feel myself becoming uncomfortable in the way that only ethical questions can make a person feel uncomfortable. I was approaching the horns of a dilemma and I sensed I would soon have to choose between the two. True, I would not be doing the procedure, since third year medical students got to do few procedures, but I knew that I would be party to any abortion that resulted from her hospitalization. So if I went along and did my share of the histories and physicals for these "TOP" assignments, there would be no making waves, no raised eyebrows. Besides, this would be the better and preferred way to get an "A" on this rotation. Or I could speak up and refuse to do this segment of the work, risk alienation, ridicule and almost certain grade reduction. I desperately wanted to compromise! Maybe there was a middle ground. And even though I wanted to take the easier road, I knew I would have an even more distasteful view of myself if I swallowed my principles and condoned the abortion. In the end, I did that which I feared to do: I nervously told the second year resident that I could not take part in any work connected with an abortion, requesting to do other work on the ward instead.

The effect of that action was profound for me. I had publicly drawn a line in the sand; I had taken a stand against abortion. But as much as it gave me some clarity, it also posed other questions. I began to think on contraception again. Specifically, if abortion was wrong, why was it wrong? And which methods of birth control were acceptable and which were not? Given my reluctance to seek any in-depth treatment of these issues by the church, it is no surprise that I felt that I would be better off just to study and think on these issues by myself. That way I wouldn't make any waves. I didn't realize that the person for whom I was afraid to make waves wasn't the people I worked with and lived with, so much as it was for me. (I know now that this was the height of pride — I didn't want to hear what anyone else had to say

on this subject; I wanted to be free to work this out for myself, in my own way, and reaching my own conclusions. In
short, I wanted to define the game, the rules and the method
of keeping score. It was a convenient way to make sure that
the game came out the way I wanted it to. The trouble is, as I
later came to accept, it is God's game!) Even so, as I struggled
with myself, I came up with what I thought was a strong
principle on which I could rest my burdened conscience: all
methods that prevented conception were morally okay, but
those that injured or killed a baby once it was conceived,
even at the two cell stage, were evil. Thus I made definitions
of convenience that allowed tubals, vasectomies, condoms,
diaphragms, spermacides, coitus interruptus (withdrawal)
and most hormonal pills, but did not allow the IUD, which I
was convinced caused early abortions. Thus I for once knew
ahead of time what I would have to do if ever asked to insert
an IUD or pressured to counsel for one. I took some comfort
in that. And besides, I could still be "for" most forms of birth
control and only "against" a few. Certainly any reasonable
person would allow me that prerogative!

Once again this classification answered some questions
for me, but it also raised others that continued to gnaw at me
and allow my uneasiness to persist, when I longed to put this
issue to rest. What about birth control pills? Don't they have
another mode of action, other than suppression of ovulation?
Do they always suppress ovulation? And once again I chose
to follow the path to truth that allowed only me to interpret
the highway signs and to make the choices about which forks
in the road to take and which to leave behind untrod. And so
I made for myself another definition of convenience: combination birth control pills were okay (since surely they prevented ovulation), but progestin-only pills were not, because
they might allow ovulation to occur (and then, conceivably, a
conception, which might be aborted even before it had a
chance to take root in the lining of the uterus). I was glad I
could make this distinction, since I could then still call myself
"pro-life." But I prayed that I would never be challenged by a
patient or a colleague to endorse or prescribe the "mini-pill,"
(progestin-only pill). And, of course, my prayers were not

completely answered. However, by the time it became an issue for patients, I was versed well enough in "medical-talk"
to counter any objections with a related scientific fact (often
only an opinion, however), and a dose of reassurance. Although I knew that ours is an increasingly consumer-wise
population, I never encountered someone who wished to
press the issue beyond my initial response. Thank God! (or so
I thought. . . now I wonder if I would have come to the truth
earlier if I had been placed in the uncomfortable position of
being challenged.)

It wasn't until I had been in private practice for ten years
that I felt the rumblings of my conscience stirring again. By
that time I had already learned how to do vasectomies and
post-partum tubal ligations (for which there was a significant
turf battle waged at the local hospital for the right of a family
physician to perform this surgery). I enjoyed this type of surgery and thought I was quite good at it. I made it a point to
do every tubal or vasectomy that I could, and I did quite a
few. I also had written countless prescriptions for birth control pills. I even fitted occasional diaphragms, although there
was really not much demand for this type of contraception in
my locale. But at the same time, I was becoming more heavily
involved with sex talks to the fifth grade boys in Osceola
County. I had been involved with this outreach for at least 10
years by this time, each year learning more and more about
how to be effective in speaking to this challenging group of
youngsters. These sessions were taking on a decidedly more
proactive stand toward abstinence. At the same time, thanks
to my partner Walt Larimore, I began to be more open about
my faith and to feel less awkward and embarrassed when
praying for and with patients. He encouraged me and challenged me to address this personal and private area of our
patients' lives. I felt like I had received a Baptist-Catholic
transfusion, but it really was just a concretizing of the faith
that I loved.

Accompanying this interest in "letting my light shine"
was an openness to feed and nourish this facet of my life.
One of the opportunities that came my way was an invitation

to attend the first Physician Conference sponsored by Focus on the Family and held at their new facility in Colorado Springs, Colorado. The theme of the conference was "Balancing Faith, Family & Practice." It was an absolutely delightful conference and a great source of encouragement for me to be with other physicians and spouses of faith for four days, learning and encouraging one another. One of the pleasant surprises of the conference was the presence of Dr. James Dobson himself. While he spoke only briefly, as I recall, he made himself available to those attending by standing at the back of the conference room to shake hands and answer questions. It was my desire to meet this great man that I had come to know and respect from his many writings and broadcasts. In fact, I wanted to get his picture — taken between my wife Cleta and myself — so I (I am slightly embarrassed to say.) could brag to my friends that I met Jim Dobson (and perhaps embellish the story a bit, too)! We shared that desire with the couple in front of us in line and so we were prepared when they asked us if we wouldn't mind taking their picture with Dr. Dobson, too. What I wasn't prepared for was what followed. When his turn came to greet Dr. Dobson, he asked the following question while posing this situation: I am greeted in the office by a sixteen year old girl whom I know to be sexually active and who is there to request birth control pills. Understanding that if I give her the pills, I'll be condoning her actions, but if I do not, she might go on to get pregnant, or worse yet, have an abortion, what should I do?

James Dobson answered him in this way: "I wouldn't presume to tell you what to do, since you are the one who knows so much more about the situation: the emotional, medical, financial context to name a few. But having said that, I know that someone, somewhere, somehow must stand up for the truth. Unless she hears the truth, how can she be expected to respond to it? The truth deserves to be told. Who is the one to speak the truth?"

When I heard the words, they pierced my heart like a sword! I knew that he was right. I knew, too, that I was the one who was supposed to speak the truth. Patients come to me not to get popular answers, but truthful answers. And they expect me to clear up confusion in their minds about all sorts of things from hypertension to allergy. Why not birth control? Where else can I expect them to hear the truth about premarital relations? And if I don't consider these issues, weigh the important aspects of these problems, and search out the truth in complicated issues, what use has my medical education and training been? The words of Matt 5:13 came to me: "It is no longer good for anything, except to be thrown out and trampled underfoot by men."

The conference ended on Sunday. My head was full of all the great ideas that I had heard and discussed. My wife too was aglow with joy about the special four days. It put a spark back in our relationship. We were excited — glad to be married, happy to be in medicine, enthused about how we might be a help to my practice, our church and our town. We couldn't wait to see our friends. On the airplane trip back to Florida, however, I couldn't get James Dobson's words out of my head: "Someone has to stand up for the truth." So, somewhere between Colorado Springs and Orlando, I resolved not to prescribe birth control pills to unmarried women. I was sure it was the right thing to do. And for once I came to a moral decision after receiving input from an outside source (albeit a very brief encounter).

I knew I would be tested on this decision I had made, but I had no idea how quickly I would be tested. They say that God moves slowly and in mysterious ways, but I found out He could move quickly and be very, very plain about His intentions. The very first morning I saw patients in the office, one was a young unmarried female. I think the only thing that distinguished her from the hypothetical situation brought up in Colorado Springs was the fact that she was 15 years old. So now the test was upon me. I swallowed hard, said an ever-so-quick prayer, took a deep breath and proceeded to tell her "No!" and why. I don't remember what I said, but just remember that I tried and then at some point realized I had spoken enough and it was time for her reaction. I feared many things. I thought she would reject my reasons; I thought she would protest; I feared she would think I was judgmental; I feared her mother would be incensed that I had refused to write a prescription and had wasted her time and money. None of these things happened. In fact, it was apparent that she accepted what I had to say and so did her mother. I was surprised! And relieved.

Other situations arose in the ensuing weeks. And probably I became better at explaining this "new" advice within the 5 to 10 minutes that I would usually spend on going over how to take the pill and the dangerous side effects/contraindications of the pill. One situation I particularly remember, however, involved a male, aged 25 or so. He came for treatment of what turned out to be an STD, probably chlamydia. After I took the cultures, a challenge was posed to me. It came from the spiritual realm. I realized I was in a position to influence this man with the implications of his behavior or I could ignore those social and spiritual consequences and just treat his body and the disease that he had contracted and was threatening to pass on. I knew that to just take the latter course would be to be like all the other doctors who would treat this as a disease in a person, not as a person with a disease. I sensed he deserved more than that. Once again I said a lightening quick prayer, took a deep breath and proceeded to point out to him his destructive behavior and its consequences. This time I inquired about what he wanted for his life and voiced my opinion that if he wanted to change that, he could. Once again I was fearful. I was afraid that this time for sure this handsome, self-assured, man-about-town would surely reject my concerns as irrelevant or pious. I was waiting for his "Yes, but. . ." answer, or worse, his indignation. I felt it coming. When he spoke, I was astounded! He said: "Thank you!" I was surprised. He almost knocked me off my feet. I never expected that sort of answer. I felt like saying thank you myself and almost did, but before I could, he continued "No one has ever talked with me before in that way." In his eyes I saw gratitude. I wonder what he saw in mine. I never saw him again after that.

While I was going through this metamorphosis toward abstinence, I was blessed to have a partner who allowed me to share with him these steps of boldness I was making. He encouraged me and allowed me to debrief about these things. But, good friend that he is, he challenged me too (even though he, at the time, was not yet convinced of these things). At one of our coffee break conversations he inquired how was it that some Catholics could accept some teachings of the Catholic Church but not others. As he asked, he also noted that it seemed proper to him that if a person wished to join a particular denomination that he should first inquire what the tenets of that denomination might be and then if he was willing to accept these, that he could join and be 100% part of that denomination. My response was that we have some Catholics who still call themselves Catholics but respectfully excuse themselves from endorsing, much less following, all the tenets of the Catholic Church — we call these people "cafeteria Catholics" — they pick and choose what they like, and still try to stay within the same general framework. But even as I said so, I felt uneasy about the concept and even a bit embarrassed that some followers of Catholicism would act that way. I soon realized that, in truth, that was exactly what I was doing when I did not accept the teaching of the Catholic Church on artificial contraception. It bothered my conscience, but not enough for me to do anything about it. I decided to just let it slide for the time being, promising myself to revisit this issue, and slide away it did. For awhile, that is.

About this time too I began to ask myself questions about the meaning of chastity for the unmarried. Did this mean no intercourse before marriage? Of course! Did it mean that God was against pleasure? No, or at lease I was pretty sure it didn't mean that. God is for pleasure, right? But, just in marriage, right? Well then, why was it that God does not allow this pleasure outside of marriage, but just as soon as the marriage ceremony is over, God endorses sex all the time? It all seemed too black and white. There seemed to be a piece of the puzzle missing. And what about contraception within marriage? How could we as adults expect our teenagers to be chaste before marriage if right after marriage we were allowed to have no restrictions on our sexual activity? It

seemed like the call to be chaste and in control of our passions was just being promoted to our younger members in
society, but immediately upon exchanging vows all this was
not applicable. There had to be more to self-mastery than
this. Weren't the maturest members of our society to be
looked to for having developed the virtues to their highest
form? This is certainly true for other adult endeavors, such as
athletics, business and leadership. Why shouldn't this also be
true of chastity? Heaven knows we need leaders in this
arena. But who was going to lead by example? Where were
those who would boldly stand up and do what was right
both in their public and their personal life?

Directly or indirectly these questions led me to Natural
Family Planning. I, of course, had heard of this before, but
what I was reading now promoted NFP as an answer to the
question of marital chastity (*Marriage is For Keeps; The Art of
Natural Family Planning.*) Furthermore, it answered what was
for me a very poignant question: How does a couple build
and maintain respect over the course of a lifetime? The question had become all the more poignant, even urgent, because
around that time, several couples that I cared for in my practice were contemplating — even threatening — divorce. This
grieved me deeply. I had known each of them separately and
as a couple; I knew their children; I had even delivered the
latest of their children. Their struggles severely affected them
and brought them to the brink of despair, but their struggles
also affected me. If I liked and respected each of them separately, why couldn't they? Why couldn't they live together
peaceably? Couldn't they see that divorce was a poor solution to their troubles? And was guaranteed to spawn other
problems that would further agonize them?

But I knew that these problems did not crop up over-
night. I was quite sure that the seeds of their problems began
a while back, even possibly, a great while back. The disagree-
ments, the arguing, the inability to forgive, the insistence that
progress could only be made if one side was first acknowl-
edged to be right — all these stumbling blocks had their ori-
gins back when the road was less rocky. There had to be
something about the early courtship and/or marriage that al-

lowed for easy resolution of these sorts of problems that was just as surely lacking in the later years of marriage. That something, it seemed to me, was loss of respect. The day they no longer looked to and on each other with respect, was the day their relationship and their marriage starting dying. It seemed logical to me then that if they could see the beauty that each of them possessed that their respect could be recouped, rekindled, and reclaimed. Marital chastity, with periodic abstinence and unity of spirit, seemed to be the way to maintain that respect once it was reestablished.

All these thoughts were circulating in my head at one time or another when I met a new patient, named Dana Lovelace. At the time of our first appointment, she was single, mid-twenties and came to my office for a physical exam. Although reluctant to ask questions about sexual activity, I forced myself this time (just because I thought I should inquire into all areas of normal adult functioning.) To my surprise she told me she was a virgin and wished to remain that way till she was married, although she had no one special in her life at that time. I tried not to register my surprise and stammered something about choosing the best path and that's how everyone in her situation should be. But because of that hurried affirmation of her own witness, I remembered her visit and a special atmosphere of trust arose out of that situation. It wasn't too much later that she came for another appointment and announced that she had indeed met someone special and was hopeful for the future. A third appointment followed some months later, this time again for a Pap smear and she announced that she was engaged to be married. I was pleased for her and rejoiced with her that God had brought this special person into her life. She had come to this office visit with a special concern on which she wanted my personal and professional opinion. She asked me which of all the methods of family planning did I consider the best, not just in terms of effectiveness, but also for her marriage. My answer came after a short pause: NFP. I shared with her why and she shared her gratitude. Although I was sure she was unaware of the effect she had on me, I mark that incident to this day as a turning point in my NFP conversion. It was the first time I had to witness about what was going on inside my head to a third party, besides my wife and myself. For my ears to hear the answer that my lips gave was every bit as convicting to me as my refusal to be a part of the medical school abortions. I had said it — now I have to live it!

But at the same time, as each step along the way called for its own courage or its own decision, each step likewise became a source of joy to me as I contemplated the pleasure it gave me to speak the truth, unfettered, unambiguously and uncompromised. Such was the effect for me of proclaiming NFP best for her marriage. It was not long after that, that I was moved to write a letter to all my patients, wherein I advised them of my decision to not prescribe artificial contraception to my patients. I was fearful of what effect it would have on these women, but the joy of speaking the truth enabled me to proceed and not count the cost. I realized, too, that this action of mine would impact my partners. (I had two other partners at that time.) So I sought and received their permission to send my letter to all the female patients in the office between the ages of 15 and 55. In all, I probably sent out 1500, greeting and signing each one. Talk about writer's cramp! And it didn't improve my handwriting either!

[Doctor Hartman's letter is reproduced in Appendix II.]

I was ready for whatever would come, I thought. I was sure there would be disappointment, muted rejection, hurt feelings, and distance in our doctor-patient relationship. Loss of income and market share were considerations, but this was not as great a fear since I knew my partners would not be joining me in my stand. What I got was not what I expected. One representative letter went as follows:

> *Dear Dr. Hartman,*
>   *Well, good for you! I am so proud to have you as our family doctor. There are not many men who have the guts to stand up for what they believe in — especially when it may affect their pocketbooks!*

There were many other letters. One was from Kentucky, where a woman wrote in support of my stand after she heard of my letter through a friend who was visiting her sister, a patient of mine. Another even came from someone on whose husband I had performed a vasectomy some years back, to say she was now pregnant and thrilled!

Of all the nearly 20 replies I got in writing and the 20 or so more I received in person, not one was hostile or angry. A few, but not many, were from Catholics. Far from being a negative force in my practice of medicine, "the letter" — as some people still refer to it — has been a source of encouragement to me. And as before, I have experienced joy from this decision, and its aftermath.

My conversion process began with my rejection of the Catholic Church's teaching on birth control and ended with my letter fully accepting her teaching against all forms of artificial contraception. I now consider myself fully Pro-Life and even like to think that's what NFP really stands for. To that end I have traveled to Omaha, Nebraska, to become a certified Natural Family Planning Medical Consultant. As such I consider myself as a resource person to people of all faiths and walks of life who wish to follow any of the several methods of NFP. My wife too has become versed and certified in NFP and actively teaches couples in Kissimmee and the surrounding areas. We have found that not only is it a great service for my patients and other couples, but it has been a source of great bonding between the two of us. It is our hope that others will pick up the challenge and follow this path. The harvest is great, but the laborers are few.

In closing, I would like to just briefly state what I consider to be the take home message of my story.

1. There are very few, if any, coincidences in life.
2. Many times, we are completely unaware of the effect we may have on other peoples' lives and actions.
3. Just hearing ourselves take a stand has the effect of dramatically reinforcing that stand.
4. Trust and obey the Lord — understanding will follow, not vice-versa.
5. That which seems the most distasteful can bring the most delight.

Indeed, the stone which the builders rejected has become the cornerstone: the Church's teaching on artificial birth control and on human sexuality was at one time the mark for me that the Church was out of touch with the modern world. Now it has become a profound source of wisdom not only for myself in my marriage relationship, but also foundational in my work as a doctor, placed here by the Divine Physician Himself to minister to His people.

I hope my story has been of some use to you. It has been good for me to tell it.

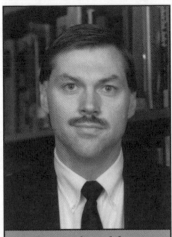

THANK YOU, JESUS, FOR HEALING ME

George E. Jay, MD

Dr. Jay graduated from medical school in 1984, having attended Mayo in Rochester, Minnesota, and completed a residency in family practice at the University of North Dakota.

He has been in a group practice — Steven's Community Medical Center in Morris, Minnesota, for eleven years. Dr. Jay considers his family his greatest honor. He and his wife Joan are parents of five children, ages 5 to 15 — Mary, Christopher, Timothy, Anthony and Nicholaus.

As a physician I always considered myself pro-life. I evangelized against abortion both before and after I became a physician. As a "pro-lifer," I was always puzzled by the fact that many pro-life activists talked about an intrinsic or built-in link between contraception and abortion. I thought because I couldn't see this link, it must not exist.

The Appointment

It was a warm day at my physician office in Morris, Minnesota. I had been a physician in a group family practice setting for over two years, and I was comfortable handling difficult situations. It was a beautiful day. The window in my medical office was open, the sun was shining, and the birds outside were singing. I was busy and my nurse Ruth was telling me to pick up the pace, because, although our schedules were already full, we had to take additional patients, as they were acutely ill. Little did I know that later that day a situation would arise that would eventually shake my practice of medicine and my personal life as it had never been shaken before.

Walking into the exam room I saw a mother and her young daughter. This was their first time in my office. I smiled and made some small talk. The expression on my face changed when the mother stated, in front of her daughter, "Well, my daughter recently started dating a boy and I thought I should bring her in and get her on the pill."

I couldn't believe what I was hearing. Although I'm ashamed to admit I used oral contraceptives in my practice and performed vasectomies, the mother's request caught me off guard. I looked at that girl. She was thirteen years old. I looked at her birth date on the chart. She had been twelve years old just several weeks prior

I was speechless. I started to get nauseated and could feel myself starting to both sweat and shake. I excused myself cordially, went into my private office, closed the door and started to pray. I knew what was occurring here was terribly wrong. I prayed, "What do you want, God?" In my heart Jesus responded, "You KNOW what I want! Your problem, George, is that you won't DO what I want!" The conviction was frightening, because God didn't allow me to use rationalization and other defense mechanisms. I couldn't wiggle out of this one. What in the world was I going to do? I prayed for strength to do God's will because I was a coward.

My Symptoms

As a ten-year-old "cradle-Catholic" growing up in St. Paul, Minnesota, people were beginning to talk openly about sexual matters. It was 1967 and the "virtues" of contraception were being extolled. I remember, in particular, one adolescent unwed mother telling me, out of the blue, that when she has older daughters she was going to be certain to get them started on the pill early. I wondered why she was telling this to a ten-year-old kid.

By the early 1970s, my mother and father, who had already been divorced for seven years, and had gotten back together, moved us to rural Cambridge, Minnesota. During my high school years, either the anti-life evangelists hadn't infiltrated our school yet, or I wasn't paying close enough attention in class to pick it up. I suspect it was a little of both.

However, the religion classes at that time were another story. They weren't really false teaching; they simply lacked substance. There was the admonition to "be nice" but with no real explanation of why. I do not recall being taught anything about sin or Hell. I didn't know if the Church taught the real presence of Christ in the Eucharist. I wasn't taught the necessity of confessing my sins to the priest. Some people sarcastically refer to this as "kumbaya catechesis." As a rebellious ninth grader I knew these religion classes were a waste of my time and I left them for the rest of my adolescence. This was a "head start" for me losing my faith later in college.

Going off to the University of Minnesota at Duluth in the mid-1970s was an exciting adventure. The anti-life evangelism seemed to get worse, with me eventually joining in the anti-life chorus, although I wouldn't have seen it that way at the time. I remember reading "the fetus will defeat us" on the bathroom wall during my freshman year. There was lots of talk of deforestation and pollution, mixed with a heavy dose of depopulation teachings. There was never a word taught about natural family planning or openness to life in the context of marriage. Tragically, I lost my faith early in college.

During my senior year, I met my wife Joan. She was the woman of my dreams. I couldn't wait to introduce her to my parents. Her shyness and the purity she radiated attracted me to the point where I actually tried to keep away from her, for HER sake! I couldn't stop thinking about her. I still can't. I didn't want her to fall for a guy like me, and I told her that after I tried to skip out on our first date, Sunday Mass. Thanks to Joan's gentle persuasion, I ended up keeping that date. Joan continues to pray tirelessly for my ongoing conversion. Praise God.

In 1980 I was off to medical school at Mayo in Rochester, Minnesota. Although Joan had been accepted into an optometry program, she decided to get a job at Mayo with her biology background and hold off on her optometry career. Joan and I wanted to see if we had a future together. We were married about a year later. More so in order to avoid drugs and potential side effects, rather than obedience to Church teaching, we decided to use natural family planning in our marriage.

In medical school, the anti-life evangelization was more intense. Several other medical students and I thought of ourselves as pro-life. Some of our verbal battles as medical students were quite intense. Looking back, I realize we weren't really pro-life, so much as we were anti-abortion. Nobody that I knew spoke out against contraception.

It was taken for granted that all would accept contraception and, do you know what? It seems everybody did. There were other anti-life moments too. Some were dramatic, some were not. I remember I was emotionally struck when a female OB/GYN specialist, teaching us a unit on embryology, kept referring to developing babies as appearing more "humanoid," as if that's not what baby developing humans are supposed to look like. When we used animal specimens in study, she never referred to a chicken fetus as "chicken-oid." I was afraid to speak up. I was "chicken-oid."

In the family practice residency at the University of North Dakota, I appreciated the instructors asking residents if we wanted to insert IUDs or avoid that on moral grounds, knowing full well that IUDs are abortifacient (can cause babies to die in the womb). I remember a fellow resident who also refused to do IUDs. I'll call him Pat. The funny thing about "Pat" was that he was a self-proclaimed atheist. During supper one evening with Pat, I impulsively asked him: "Pat, I'm pro-life. I can understand why I don't want to use IUDs in my practice. But you, you're an atheist. Why don't you, of all people, feel free to just go ahead and use them?" Pat replied, "Even as an atheist, I can see that it's just not right to kill your fellow-man, no matter what stage of development he or she is at in his/her lifetime."

I was awestruck and dumbfounded. Here was this self-proclaimed atheist who wasn't using IUDs because he thought it was intrinsically wrong. I went away wondering how all these other doctors could insert IUDs, knowing full well the IUDs abortifacient potential, while claiming Jesus was Lord over their lives? I was too cowardly to ask.

I still cringe when I read Ezekiel 33:7-9 (also Ez. 3:16-19) and other verses that implore us to give appropriate warning to people. After we remove the log from our own eyes, Jesus doesn't tell us to go and relax. He says then go and tell your brother his fault (c.f. Matt. 7:5, Luke 6:42). God have mercy on me for my lack of courage in admonishing my fellow sinners.

Meanwhile, Joan picked up her Master's degree in speech pathology at the University of North Dakota. She is trained to help people with their speech difficulties. She has worked with post-stroke patients, children who stutter or have word pronunciation problems, etc. This led to our discussion of which one of us would undergo mutilation. Would I have a vasectomy or would Joan undergo a tubal ligation? Fortunately, this never occurred, but sad to say, it was discussed and accepted in the heart.

As Lent approached in 1986, I remember getting upset with Joan's suggestion that we have a three or four minute family prayer time daily during Lent. My point was that we go to Mass on Sunday, said prayers before meals, and Joan and I prayed briefly together before bed. I gave in to Joan's request, and our daily family prayer life has since blossomed tremendously.

I'm sure our children are one of the main ways God has worked on both Joan and I. After residency, we traveled to a private practice on the prairies of western Minnesota, where I currently practice in Morris. Between medical school and residency, Joan and I had three boys and after we located to Morris, we have since had another boy and a little girl. As we had more children, it seems we took our faith more seriously. I mean it's one thing if I was struggling spiritually, but Joan and I wanted better for our children. We hope and pray that God will bless us with more children.

My Diagnosis

Two years into my practice I encountered the situation with the thirteen-year-old girl and her mother. I couldn't believe that this mother was facilitating an illicit sexual relationship with her own daughter and her new boyfriend. Was I going to facilitate the betrayal of the child as well?

I went into my private office and prayed for wisdom and courage. As I went back into the patient exam room, although I thought I knew what I was going to say, I still wasn't sure if I could. Do you remember as a child, holding your nose, closing your eyes, and jumping into the deep end of the pool for the first time? Well, that's how I felt.

I told the mother, in front of her daughter, "I have decided that for a variety of reasons this child should not be involved in a sexual relationship and should not be taking oral contraceptives. There will be no charge for today's visit. I hope you will take my recommendations to heart." The mother was shocked.

She told me that she was a "paying customer" and that I HAD to do this. I told her I did not have to do this, and was not going to play in this. I reminded her that there was no charge for the visit. At this, although she was still indignant, she left the office visibly upset. Ironically, her daughter appeared relieved.

This episode started me thinking about the contraceptive issue in more detail. Unfortunately, it didn't change my prescribing habits. I still used oral contraceptives on women in my practice, but I knew I had to spend time thinking, praying, and reading on this issue.

Things went on this way until my wife's mother, Rita, came to live with us for a few months while recovering from colon cancer surgery and multiple post-operative complications. Rita had many tubes, fistulae, and much pain. With Joan's mother — a very humble, prayerful, and holy woman — living with us, we were forced to think often of eternal things and much less about worldly goods. About this time,

Joan and I heard about people making religious pilgrimages in Europe and we decided to take Rita on one. I suppose we always held out hope for a miraculous cure, but we thought that even if Rita were not cured, she would be bolstered spiritually. Ironically, it was the cancer eating away at her that actually seemed to "bolster" her. I recall asking Rita one day, "Who are you offering up your sufferings for?" This question caught me more off guard then it did Rita. She calmly answered, "my children." I asked Rita to offer up some of her sufferings for me as well. She said she would.

Several months before our pilgrimage, I did a couple of other things I had not done before. I struggled to fast in order to open my heart to God's graces in a fuller way to obey Jesus' statement that His disciples will fast (c.f. Mark 2:20, Matt. 6:16 and 9:15). I also read the four Gospels — Matthew, Mark, Luke and John. We continued to prepare to take Rita on this spiritual pilgrimage, which was now just several months away, not knowing that Rita would be too sick to go when the time came.

Although I don't deliver babies, I had and have a busy office GYN practice. I always considered myself pro-life, and had never used Depo-Provera shots because I heard in residency that this preparation was abortifacient. I never considered the birth pill control an abortifacient. I suppose if I had known that the oral contraceptive pill was potentially abortifacient, I would have had to cross the contraceptive issue earlier in my career, but I was perfectly happy in my self-imposed ignorance. No one in medical school or my residency brought up the question. I suspect there are many people like me who want to consider themselves pro-life, but really are not. We adopted the cowardly "don't ask, don't tell" attitude in training about whether or not "the pill" was abortifacient. We didn't do much to try to uncover the mystery either.

One morning, as I was getting out of my vehicle in the parking lot at the hospital, I met a pharmaceutical representative. I was in a hurry and didn't want to spend much time with him. When he began talking about a new product that was available, my interest perked up. The product was an implantable birth-control device called Norplant. I had already read about Norplant in the medical journals and I couldn't wait to give it a try in my practice. This was my chance to find out more about Norplant. Recall, I considered myself pro-life.

I asked the pharmaceutical representative if this Norplant was abortifacient. Pharmaceutical representatives know your name, face and practice habits. The drug-rep looked and smiled and said, "Well, yes, it is potentially abortifacient, but the chances are small, about the same chance of inducing an abortion as the oral contraceptives that you already use in your practice." He quoted me a percentage, but I didn't respond. I was too busy feeling the proverbial knife that was just thrust into my now-broken heart. Could I have been playing a role in potentially killing babies all along? Why hadn't I tried to answer this question before for myself? Why haven't I at least asked someone? Why didn't I do some reading? How many babies died at my (prescribing) hands? Could this be true?

Internally I was a mess. I smiled at the drug-rep, made some small talk, and excused myself. I decided to do my hospital rounds later and went straight to my office to review my GYN textbook sources to try to answer this "unanswerable dilemma." It took me about four minutes of reading to confirm what the drug-rep told me. It was true! Oral contraceptives were potentially abortifacient! Now what was I going to do? I certainly didn't want to kill off any babies. Even if there was only a small chance, that is substantial. How would I tell Joan about this? My ignorance was certainly not excusable, as it was not just laziness, but a reluctance to explore these truths prior to being challenged by what the drug-rep told me. I couldn't claim my conscience led me to the fact that "dishing out" oral contraceptives was OK either.

The Cure

When it came time for our pilgrimage, Rita was too sick to go. She eventually passed away later that year from complications. I was wrestling with the whole contraceptive issue during our pilgrimage. I had been fasting, praying, reading Sacred Scripture, and thinking of my dilemma. My biggest self-argument was that if these people didn't contracept, they would commit a worse sin, that of abortion. I reasoned I was saving lives, but part of me responded "you can't accomplish good by doing evil." (c.f. Romans 3:8) I knew that my first calling was for ME to be a faithful servant of God. Only after removing the log in my eye, could I give an effective witness for truth. My first calling was to worry about my obedience. Then I could worry about other people's disobedience. God's grace works through truth, and in spite of falsehood. I wanted God to work through me, instead of have to work in spite of me.

During our pilgrimage, there were long lines for confession. I think I prepared myself well for confession. I was told of a very gifted confessor who our group leader had gotten to know over the years. He was from France, but happened to be in the country we were visiting. I heard of the many gifts of this humble, quiet, thin young man who was to hear our confessions. This priest heard confessions for hours. When it was around midnight he was leaving and I still hadn't had my confession heard. I was told he might be back the following day. I had heard that this priest, when getting home to the family he was staying with, would spend many hours every night in front of the Blessed Sacrament. He certainly didn't sleep much. Fortunately, he was back the next day, hearing confessions again. When it was almost my turn, I still had some hardness of heart and was somewhat impenitent. My attitude was "Well, I'll get this and ALL my sins my whole life long out in the open, and then we will see what happens." Even as I prepared for confession, I had not yet decided to give up using contraceptives in my practice.

It was mid-afternoon and my turn for confession finally came. I heard some pretty awesome stories from some of the people that were coming out of the confessional, a makeshift place in a room of one of the local families that lived in this mountainous area. Here I was giving my confession to this priest and was surprised when I looked at him. He was on his knees praying! I could hear little quiet whispers occasionally from him. I'm thinking something between, "Well, this is easy. He's not even paying attention." and "What a joker! I'm wasting my time as this priest isn't even listening to me." He even had his eyes closed. I remember feeling like I was confessing my sins to the wall, so I just stopped in the middle of my confession. His eyes slowly opened and he directed me to go on.

Soon after, I stalled again in giving my confession, thinking I was again confessing to the wall. At this point, he must have known what I was thinking because he paused to converse with me regarding my confession and it was obvious to me now that he not only heard my confession, but assimilated what I told him very well. I went on. I thought of myself as all done with my confession, but he asked me to go on. Then, the priest started to tell me my sins that I hadn't confessed, and told me of a sin I had committed. At first, I didn't remember it and I denied the sin. Later he reminded me of this sin and gave me more specific details. I still didn't remember it and was a little upset that he brought it up again after I had specifically denied it. The confession went on and he reminded me a third time of this sin. Only this time he gave many details surrounding the event. As I was about to indignantly deny this again, I remembered with complete clarity the episodes that he was reminding me of. Tears of repentance welled up not just in my eyes, but seemed to be welling up from the depths of my being.

As Father gave me absolution, I could feel the power of Christ's blood, cleansing me in a new way. I was feeling the very first gift the risen Lord gave to the apostles in the upper room that first Easter night as He breathed on them, "If you forgive the sins of any, they are forgiven; if you retain the sins of any, they are retained." (John 20:23) I was on the receiving end of Christ's promised outpouring of the Holy Spirit. I didn't know it at the time that sorrow for my sins, or contrition, was required for the sacrament of reconciliation to be valid. While I wasn't contrite before the confession, I certainly received that grace during the confession. Father could see my contrition and subsequently gave me absolution and a penance.

When I got out of the confessional, I was set free. My whole outlook and attitude had changed from "Well, I'll get it out there in the confessional and we'll see what happens," to "I am set free." My only regret about the whole contraceptive issue is that I had betrayed Jesus in the first place. Never again would I be using contraception in my medical practice or anywhere else. Another physician on the trip came to the same conclusion.

I thought about what they were going to say back in Morris in the clinic and around town. You know what? I didn't care. I thought to myself, "I will not be intimidated." Joan was very supportive as well and this also helped, but I knew that making this choice was only part of my journey.

I was somewhat unprepared for the reaction I received when I returned to Morris. When I got back to the clinic, I explained to my nurse, the staff, and my colleagues what my intentions were. I was absolutely floored when my physician colleagues passively supported me in my decision. I recommended abstinence to unmarried patients who wanted oral contraceptives renewed, and talked to married couples about openness to life or natural family planning (NFP). I explained that with NFP there are times of abstinence, just as there are times of abstinence in all relationships. When husbands and wives are apart, they abstain. Husbands and wives abstain when they go out in public. I lost some patients, but actually gained other patients as well, and continue to have a busy medical practice.

In addition to acceptance from my physician colleagues, I was pleasantly surprised to find many Bible-alone Christians who either supported me or said "although I don't agree with you, I really respect you for being able to live out such a counter-cultural teaching in today's world."

Just as I had some pleasant surprises, there were some unpleasant ones too. The unpleasant experiences often came from sources I wouldn't have expected to be in opposition to Church teaching. Some Catholic friends and family members, and even official representatives of the Catholic Church, disagreed with my decision. My brother Jon, who is a sharp attorney, challenged me on the contraceptive issue. I asked him to prayerfully study the subject. He accepted, I think, with the idea that not only would he be able to refute the Church's position, but bring me "back" as well. After several months into his study, he and his wife Theresa concluded the Church was right! Later, Jon had his vasectomy reversed. Some months after the reversal, I remember seeing Theresa holding their new son Joseph, tears welling up in her eyes. Theresa told me, "without submitting to the Church, we would not have been graced with this sweet precious child." Then she gave her son a motherly embrace. More tears of joy flowed from her and Jon as well. They are evangelists for the Catholic faith, and since have had two more children and are expecting another.

My wife Joan enjoys sharing the Church's teachings on the contraceptive issue, too. Joan has been a constant source of encouragement to me since this conversion of heart. Joan and Theresa both say some of their most intense moments are when sharing an "openness-to-life position as God's will" with other moms, in the kitchen over juice and coffee. Both Joan and Theresa sprinkle their ministries with much prayer every week in front of the Blessed Sacrament — worshipping Jesus Himself in the Flesh. They both also ask our spiritual mother, the Blessed Virgin Mary, to intercede on behalf of those they are evangelizing.

The Prognosis

I've met some very good and faithful priests regarding this issue and I can't say enough about them. I recently attended a large physicians' meeting and was addressed by a young priest who told us "there is an army of young priests coming up who affirm all the Faith including *Humanae Vitae.* Just hang on! We support the Pope and subject ourselves to his authority." How very reassuring

Our own parish priest, Father Gerald Dalseth, challenged his congregation in a homily on Ezekiel 33:7 to "respect, reassess and submit to the church's teachings on *Humanae Vi-*

tae." My wife and I cried tears of joy. After Mass many came up and gave Father encouragement for his words.

A Prescription

I pray, fast and read the bible and the **Catechism**. I want to keep the faith now that I have discovered these truths. Some personal favorites always encourage me: Scott and Kimberly Hahn, Human Life International's Father Marx, Steve Wood and Karl Keating. I depend upon John Kippley's superb book, **Birth Control and Christian Discipleship**, along with anything written by Father Hardon, to both strengthen me and help me bring this truth to others. Janet Smith's tape "CONTRACEPTION: Why Not?" and excellent Catholic magazines, for example *Envoy* and *This Rock*, are other helpful sources to me.

Joan and I have become Natural Family Planning instructors, which we see as an important stronghold in the pro-life battle. Finally, I draw the most strength from just embracing the sacraments, and remembering why God gave us marriage in the first place: to have spouses help each other get to heaven and to present godly offspring to God. Confident of the goodness of His plan, it is easy for me to understand and follow the Church's teaching on contraception.

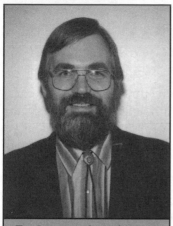

FROM THE DARKNESS OF DECEPTION TO THE LIGHT OF TRUTH

Stanley Lang, M.D.

Dr. Lang graduated in 1978 from the University of Kansas School of Medicine and completed his residency in Family Practice at the Southwestern Medical School in Wichita Falls, Texas.

For the past 17 years, Dr. Lang has practiced in a group family medicine center that he established, the Agape Family Health Center, located in DuBois, Pennsylvania.

Considering the roles of Husband and Father to be his greatest awards and honors, Stan and his wife Sheri have five children ranging in ages from 19 years old to 10 months — Noel, Beth, Maria, Katherine and Christopher.

I am a family physician, in practice for almost 18 years. I am in a family practice setting with other physicians who have committed to incorporating their faith into the practice of medicine.

The idea for attempting to do this grew from our residency and medical school experiences during which time we recognized the general hostility of organized medicine to the Christian faith. Initially, we experienced the need to be in practice with like-minded individuals for the purpose of being faithful in our walk with the Lord because of the relative difficulty we could encounter in a generally anti-Christian environment. This evolved to recognizing the need to incorporate spiritual ministering to our patients, both those with faith and those without. We realized that we would be better at this if we were in practice with individuals where we could encourage each other in this goal.

So it is within the backdrop of this Christian mission to integrate faith into practice that the issue of prescribing oral contraceptives arose.

One of my partners is somebody that I went to medical school with and, actually, also to high school. Over the years we had wrestled with the issue of oral contraceptives intermittently, primarily because of our fear that they were abortifacient. We had actually talked to people several times who should know and had been reassured that the pill was 100% successful in preventing ovulation. At the time we did not go back to the source documents ourselves.

After being in practice several years, one of our new partners joining us requested not to have to prescribe oral contraceptives. We permitted this and understood this to be a decision based on the possibility of the abortifacient action of oral contraceptives. During that time we were most influenced by the moral dilemma of not wanting to abandon patients who "needed" this service even if we had some personal reservations about prescribing oral contraceptives.

The OCP issue remained a back burner issue until a discussion that I had with a theologian who had been an evangelical Protestant and became a Catholic. Because I am the only Catholic in our group of Christian physicians of diverse backgrounds, I was interested in understanding how we could better grow in unity. As I discussed this question with this theologian, he immediately indicated that he believed that without tackling the issue of contraception (which I had not raised with him) and reaching unity on that, any other unity would be superficial and limited permanently in its ability to grow in depth.

After that discussion I shared these thoughts with the rest of our group of four physicians and we spent the next year attempting to discern this question. We looked at and studied *Humanae Vitae* and a book written by a Protestant showing a Protestant perspective on contraception and read some of the medical literature that demonstrates the frequency of breakthrough ovulation even on high dose birth control pills. The lower dose OCPs had substantially higher rates of break-through ovulation.

As we further looked at the action of the "morning after pill" — that is, the use of the higher dose OCPs post-coital — it seemed certain that the primary action was an endometrial effect. The other proposed "contraceptive" mechanisms of action seemed to vary between ridiculous and unlikely as primary mechanisms of action.

Focusing on the "morning-after" mechanism in light of the known breakthrough ovulation rate on regular pill use — knowing that there are both ectopic and successful uterine pregnancies on OCPs (I just had two patients who came to me for pregnancy care who had been on OCPs and had taken them correctly) — made the probability of occasional to fre-quent abortifacient action of OCPs to be beyond doubt. Nev-ertheless, we had decided that we would not as a group make any decision without being unanimous and peaceful in our unanimity.

The frequently held reason for a Christian pro-life physi-cian continuing to prescribe OCPs is that we don't have the right to impose our values on our patients. My discussion with the theologian had given me a framework to see that my responsibility was to be true to myself and not ever to partici-pate in the sinful action of another person.

Reaching this point of reasoning was sufficient for three of the partners but our fourth partner was not swayed until actually sitting down and talking with an NFP instructor. During this time the woman instructor shared many personal experiences that touched the heart of our fourth partner and in an instant his opposition, which was based on false guilt, evaporated.

We then decided to notify our patients of our decision to eliminate oral contraceptives. We decided that, publicly, we would use the abortifacient action as the main reason behind our decision. Privately, we had already concluded that the other criticisms about the effect of the contraceptive mentality on our society were also valid but decided not to use that as the basis for our public stance.

We intended to be as non-controversial as possible and quiet in presenting this information in a letter to our patients, but, for some reason, our decision was "leaked" to the newspaper so it became quite public. The local paper desired to interview us and consented to the unusual criteria that we would have final word on the final edited version of what would be printed.

We were positive that we would lose a lot of patients with this decision. In fact, we did lose the majority of our younger reproductive age females to, at least, gynecological care, although many of them stayed in the practice for other reasons.

We experienced confirmation that this was the right decision before the Lord in that there was a universal and complete lifting of an unrecognized weight for each of us as we moved away from prescribing any kind of chemical contraceptives regardless of the setting. This stance has allowed us to be consistent in our public condemnation of IVF programs that are also abortifacient and cloning research that will experiment on human embryos, and has given clarity to the evolving issue regarding the "morning after pill."

The pro-abortion attempt to redefine the beginning of pregnancy as implantation of a fertilized ovum as opposed to the fertilization of the egg is a battle that we would not have even been inclined to take on had we not been focused on the whole abortifacient issue of OCPs.

An interesting coincidence that also occurred with our decision to stop prescribing OCPs was that we were looking for many years for a Christian counselor who would fit in with the style of our practice. Within a month after stopping prescribing contraceptives, the Lord brought a Christian counselor who I believe was uniquely prepared to work in our practice.

In retrospect, the practice of prescribing contraceptives was a definite undermining effect in trying to integrate our faith into the practice of medicine. I remain very thankful to the Lord that He brought me and our group out of the bondage of prescribing contraceptives. I feel genuine sorrow for those physicians who are pro-life and know in their hearts that chemical contraceptives are abortifacient yet feel stuck because of their perception of financial constraints or other reasons of false guilt.

We decided that we would have to offer a high quality alternative to chemical contraceptives and, at the same time we decided to discontinue the chemicals, we decided to get trained in the Creighton Model of Natural Family Planning. This has been a blessing for many patients who have benefited from the unique treatment options that the Creighton Model offers. Since introducing this option we have slowly attracted patients who desire not only pregnancy care but also treatment of many of the GYN problems that the Creighton system uniquely can treat.

This transition from the contraceptive mentality to the Creighton Model program, treating both obstetrical and gynecological problems, has markedly increased my enjoyment and appreciation of OB/GYN in a family practice setting. The part of family practice that fascinated me the most as a resident in training has regained the position of being the most enjoyable treatment that I give in my daily activities.

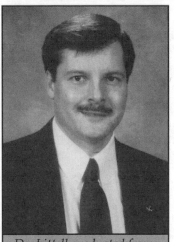

Dr. Littell graduated from the George Washington University School of Medicine in 1987 and completed a residency in family practice with the U.S. Army at Ft. Lewis in Tacoma, Washington. After four years as a faculty member with a family medicine residency program in Augusta,Georgia, Dr. Littell left the military and spent a year in emergency medicine.

Dr. Littell has practiced in Montana and Michigan and has recently joined Heritage Family Physicians, a group family practice in Kissimmee, Florida. He is a Board Member of the Catholic Medical Association and Founder and President of Family Physicians for Life, Inc. John and his wife Kathleen have three young daughters: Anne Marie, Mary Kathleen and Claire Marie.

FROM CONTRACEPTION TO NFP: ONE PHYSICIANS'S JOURNEY

John T. Littell, MD

I have been a Roman Catholic since birth, and a physician for ten years, yet I only became a truly "Catholic" physician about four years ago, while stationed at Fort Gordon, Georgia, as an Army family physician.

Prior to that time, I considered myself to be an active, "practicing" (for what?) Catholic, having spent one year living and studying at a major diocesan (Catholic) seminary following my graduation from Cornell University in 1980. I spent another year teaching high school biology at a Catholic high school, and even had the distinction of introducing a curriculum on contraception into the classroom. At the time, I thought I was doing a major service for the teenagers in my classroom, providing them with "factual" information concerning the action and efficacy of the available birth control methods. Though I stressed abstinence at the time, I clearly did not understand how much I usurped the role of the students' parents, not to mention the role of the Church, in presenting a bevy of misleading "facts" to such a captive, if not sexually active, audience.

My years of medical school (1983-1987) and residency (1987-1990) led me to an increasing understanding of my role as a "Christian" physician and person, as I became involved in Christian fellowships (often, the only Catholic member). While I was proud of the many aspects of my faith that differentiated me from my Christian, non-Catholic friends, I found myself ignoring the teachings of the Church with regards to birth control. I digested the material presented to me by my medical schoolteachers (the rhythm method as "Vatican roulette") and had no difficulty adopting the practice of vasectomy and the prescription of oral contraceptives. I chose, mostly for pragmatic reasons, not to master the technique of tubal ligation.

Following my residency, I spent four years as a faculty member in a family practice residency located at Fort Gordon, Georgia. My wife Kathleen and I had been married after my internship year, and we proceeded to have each of our three daughters while in Augusta, Georgia. As a faculty member, I enjoyed teaching medical students and residents the intricacies of prescribing oral contraceptives or performing vasectomies. I had my own "rule" which I used in screening candidates for vasectomy: patients must be married, over thirty years of age, and have at least three children. How presumptuous!

One of my major interests, even prior to medical school, is the field of medical ethics, and I have always considered myself to be actively "pro-life" in all my endeavors. Hence, when I became aware of the abortifacient properties of birth control methods such as the IUD and Norplant, I chose not to incorporate them into my practice, and tried to educate others about their life-destroying properties. When injectable, long-acting progestins became available ("Depo-Provera"), I opposed it not so much for the possible (though less likely) abortifacient properties as for the many detrimental effects it leads to in its users (e.g., osteoporosis, depression, weight gain).

My approach to patient care, at least with regards to family planning, focused on three aspects of my own practice: My Christian faith, my commitment to pro-life activity, and my firm belief in the tenet Primum non nocere — "First, do no harm." My Catholic faith was, of course, of primary importance to my marriage and family, and my wife and I had, early on, ruled out the use of artificial methods of birth control. This decision, I might add, was made as much for health reasons (we knew, in our hearts, that "the pill" was not "good" for Kathleen) as for religious reasons. Hence, three daughters in our first five years of marriage! Yet, I truly felt that I could not, as a Catholic physician, expect my patients to observe the same moral and religious code which Kathleen and I had adopted. The only setting in which I absolutely refused to prescribe birth control was for patients who were unmarried, and most emphatically, teenagers. Rather, I would spend as much time as they would allow, counseling them regarding STDs and the damaging effects and known dangers of premarital sexual relations.

In the spring of 1993, I was unexpectedly "deployed" for one weekend to St. Thomas and St. Croix, for the purpose of performing physical examinations on Army reservists living on the islands. This assignment was supposed to be a "benny," and I was allowed the option of bringing my wife along. However, Kathleen was still nursing our second daughter, and so I enjoyed the company of one of the residents from our program, Cpt. Bill Blanke (who, as it turned out, was also unable to bring his wife). During our flight to the Caribbean, I noticed a copy of *The Linacre Quarterly* in Bill's briefcase. *The Linacre* is the quarterly publication of the Catholic Medical Association. Borrowing it from Bill, I noted that one of the articles was written by Dr. Kevin Murrell, a staff psychiatrist at the Medical College of Georgia in Augusta. Upon my return from the Caribbean, I contacted Dr. Murrell, who has since become a very close friend and mentor, as will be discussed below.

Bill Blanke and I went on to discuss various aspects of our lives as Catholics, and as physicians. Bill challenged me with regards to my position on birth control: "Either you are a Catholic physician or you are not." Bill, a graduate of Creighton University, was familiar with the option of natural family planning, and did not, in his own training, prescribe artificial methods of birth control to his patients. When he challenged me to do likewise, I decided it was time to take another look at my commitment to my Catholic faith.

Returning to Atlanta, Georgia, I first contacted Dr. Murrell by phone, and was invited to attend the next meeting of the local Catholic Physicians Guild, which was held on first Saturdays. Ultimately, it was the great affirmation and encouragement that I received from this group of Catholic physicians that led me to stop prescribing artificial methods of birth control, and to explore the option of natural family planning.

My decision to refrain from prescribing oral contraceptives or other artificial means of birth control (and to stop doing vasectomies) was, as stated earlier, implemented in stepwise fashion (most likely due to my own lack of courage rather than any other supposed patient-related concerns). In seeking to learn more about natural family planning, I was pleased to discover that there were several organizations which offered instruction in NFP, i.e., CCL, Family of the Americas, BOMA, and Pope Paul VI Institute in Omaha.

With regards to teaching NFP, I need to emphasize that there are many ways to present the wonderful news about NFP to patients and fellow Catholics and Christians. "It's in the presentation," to borrow a phrase. I believe that any success I've had in introducing couples to the "alternative" of NFP is attributable to God's grace, rather than any particular effort on my part. I have been most fortunate in being exposed to just about every major school of thought with regards to NFP. Kathleen and I learned through the CCL (the Couple to Couple League) in 1993 and would have become a teaching couple with CCL were it not for their requirement that Kathleen be a "full-time" mother for the first three years of each child's life. In retrospect, that is exactly what Kathleen did for our last daughter Claire. But she wanted to at least have the option of returning to work at some point.

Since CCL did not pan out (although I continue to utilize many of their resources), I turned to Mercedes Wilson, who in turn asked whether I would serve as her "medical advisor" for Family of the Americas. Ms. Wilson, along with Dr. Hanna Klaus, was one of the original "students" of Drs. Billings in the 1960s.

While I found the materials provided by Mercedes Wilson to be excellent, I still knew that I needed to learn NFP in a more structured environment. I was unable to take the time out of my private practice schedule in Montana to take Dr. Hilgers' course at Pope Paul VI. Fortunately, I discovered "BOMA," which is the national organization that grew out of the work that Dr. Billings accomplished in the U.S.

Since Kathleen and I adopted the use of OM (the Billings Ovulation Method), we found it very easy to learn and apply. Similarly, the couples I have worked with seem pleased to find that the method is not cumbersome. Most convincingly, the OM of NFP has been taught and implemented throughout the world — even Mother Teresa required that her sisters learn the Billings Method.

During the remainder of my military service, I encountered little resistance and/or criticism concerning this shift in my practice of family medicine. For the most part, my patients were either beyond their reproductive years, or were unmarried dependents who, as stated earlier, would not receive prescriptions for contraceptives from me in any case. I had decided NOT to prescribe contraceptives for my unmarried, sexually active patients but to allow my married patients to have at least a "3-month trial period" during which I would prescribe their "last" supply of oral contraceptives, while they explored the option of NFP. Again, this decision was based upon my sincere belief that I was doing the best thing for my patients. Clearly, however, I was not yet convinced about the absolute moral imperatives that presented themselves along these lines.

After my military career, I spent one year as an emergency room physician, where I had little or no role as a provider of contraception. Of course, I did everything possible (or so I thought) to prevent unexpectedly pregnant women from exploring the option of abortion, but that is another story.

It was during my three years as a family physician in Small Town America that I first encountered significant opposition because of my views on birth control.

In northeastern Montana, where I served with the NHSC as the lone physician on call for the entire county of 2300 persons, I made it clear to my patients that I would not prescribe artificial contraceptives (continuing my lone exception of three months supply for newly married patients). I gave a brief course on NFP (though not particularly organized!) just to allow my patients an opportunity to explore this option.

Unbeknownst to me, one of my clinic nurses, and a number of other hospital personnel (including women who were prominent members of my church!) began to undermine my role in the community. A new hospital administrator chose to place his trust in these established personnel, and sent off a letter to the state of Montana in which he asserted, among other things, the following:

> *Much of [Dr. Littell's] counseling seems to hinge on his personal beliefs, birth control seems to be one of his targets and he often ties treatment of other complaints to getting birth control pills. In one case, a woman had brought her daughter in to see Dr. Littell. When he found out that the girl was on the pill, he called the boyfriend of the girl to counsel him. The boy did not know that the girl was on the pill. The mother was furious at this breech of confidentiality and related that she would sue, but that*

the intent was to have it be private. Much of the
counseling seems to be unrequested, even unwel-
come, perceived as prying.

Interestingly, the above "case" never occurred. There was no such girl, no such boyfriend, no such mother. And the hospital administrator, when confronted by me, simply related that he heard this from another source at the hospital.

The administrator had written this letter to the professional assistance program in Montana, for the purpose of initiating an investigation into my professional behavior. In the days following this letter, multiple hospital personnel, and even my own priest, related stories and perceptions to a supposedly impartial investigator, the sum total of which led to me being required to go for psychiatric counseling — or else, lose my license to practice medicine

At no time did the investigator visit with the guidance counselor at the school (where I had initiated a much-needed program for children of divorce), or the previous hospital administrator, or the many ministers, professionals, and other townspeople who ultimately rallied to keep me in this small town on the frontier of Montana. In fact, the investigation was a sham, but I was in no position to fight, for a number of reasons — not the least of which was financial. So we left Montana, and sought refuge in another town where my wife had family, in Michigan.

The entire story is too lengthy to relate here, but suffice it to say that my experience in Montana was followed up by a similar, and no less painful, experience in a somewhat larger small town in south central Michigan. Once the sole obstetrician in my new town got wind of my approach both to obstetrics (i.e., "natural childbirth") and birth control, he refused to provide obstetrical back up which was necessary for me to obtain obstetrical privileges. In essence, I was denied the right to practice obstetrics after nearly ten years of delivering babies, assisting on C-sections, etc.

Ultimately, I turned to neighboring hospitals for support, which led to even more persecution (might I use this term?)

by my own hospital personnel. Within the course of one month (January, 1998), the obstetrician and his new partner, as well as three other physicians, who, as it happened, were on the executive committee of the hospital, initiated a letter-writing campaign from patients who had either been refused contraception or were taken off artificial means of birth control by me. This was followed by a meeting in which I was threatened with loss of admitting privileges for the following reason: "Dr. Littell, you are not getting along well with other staff." In truth, I got along extremely well with those (precious few!) staff with whom my practice did not compete, and particularly those established staff members who were secure enough in their own identity and practice to accommodate a new physician with a new outlook on medicine and patient care.

My experience in this town, from which I am about to depart, can perhaps best be summed up by the following comment, which was made by the present hospital administrator to my wife and me in our "final" visit with him, "If I'd known that my wife (the administrator's wife) would have a Catholic physician after the birth of our child, I never would have let her choose him." Yes, I'm afraid to say that the persecution of Christians — and particularly, Catholics — who choose to lead their professional lives in accordance with their values and beliefs, is alive and well in these Godforsaken times.

Interestingly, and very significantly, I must add that my patients have never been a source of persecution for me in this regard. When presented with the factual information that I have accumulated over the years concerning the adverse effects of hormonal contraception, tubal ligation, etc., every one of my patients has the same response — "Why didn't my previous doctors tell me about this?" Patients are receptive to the truth, and to the option of natural family planning. I do not "shove my beliefs down their throats." I present them with options which, for the most part, they had not previously considered, and allow them to make their own truly INFORMED decisions about these most delicate and sensitive aspects of the human existence — our abilities to express our sexual selves in intimacy with our spouse, and, at the same, to allow the generative power of God to be present in the blessed act of procreation.

By and large, those who have been my detractors and persecutors are persons with little joy in their lives. Almost without exception, they have been persons who have either never known the joys of marriage and childrearing, or whose experience of abuse, divorce, and rejection leads them to exercise their influence to damage those who would attempt to interject just a bit of Christian truth, with its concomitant unspeakable happiness and peace, into the world around them. I have escaped my experiences in Montana and Michigan with my marriage intact, and indeed flourishing, and my children well adjusted, and each day rejoicing in the many gifts that their God gives to them. And, quite happily, I have had the privilege of presenting the truth to several thousand patients, and to share their smiles, as well as their tears, as they've discovered new ways of looking at their own relationships, with each other and with their Lord. What a privilege it is to be a Catholic, Christian, family physician, and to have been able to expose patients to "the way, the truth, and the life" — so that, in turn, both their lives and mine would be more fulfilled, more peaceful.

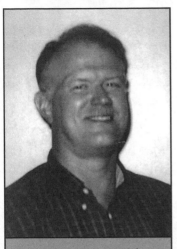

Dr. Oliver graduated from Louisiana State University Medical Center in New Orleans in 1979, and completed a residency in Family Practice, followed by a Fellowship in Obstetrics at Tallahassee Memorial Regional Medical Center in Tallahassee, Florida.

Dr. Oliver began practice in Metairie, Louisiana, and after a year, he relocated to Altha, Florida, where he spent the next five years practicing in a solo rural private practice. In 1989 he joined the faculty of the Tallahassee Medical Center Family Practice Residency Program and worked as a full-time faculty member until 1995. Dr. Oliver is currently again in private practice in Tallahassee, Florida, where he does a full scope of care including Obstetrics and Newborns.

FIRST DO NO HARM

H. Whit Oliver, MD

The practice of medicine is both enjoyable and exciting but I personally have found it to be also quite challenging. When I chose to follow the Church's teaching on family planning, I was indeed challenged, but through this decision I have been much more fulfilled in my vocation as a physician.

I became enthusiastic about natural family planning after reading a series of articles printed in the British Medical Journal in 1990-92 by Dr. Ryder, a reproductive endocrinologist. Dr. Ryder has studied and has helped prove the effectiveness of NFP in preventing pregnancy. I also discovered the World Health Organization's large population studies — across a wide range of ethnic, religious, and socio-economic backgrounds — which showed NFP being effective at levels comparable to the most ef-

Whit has been married to wife Molly since 1976, and together they have four children, Adam, Cornelia, Claire and Warren.

fective contraceptive methods, even comparable to the effectiveness of sterilization, for couples willing to have post-ovulatory intercourse only. Furthermore, these latter studies were conducted among poor and uneducated women. I was astounded! None of this information had been made available to me through years of premedical, medical, and postgraduate education. Thus I began a journey of exploration into what at first seemed to be hidden scientific data, through a questioning of the validity of all scientific fact, to an ever deepening journey of faith on which I continue today.

As background information, my wife Molly and I married in 1976. Although I had attended Mass with my wife for many years, it was not until the baptism of our third child, Claire, in 1985 that I was formally received into the Catholic Church. Molly had begun the birth control pill several months before we were married, and while she always commented on, and complained about, how she didn't feel exactly well on them, she continued with it since the pill was considered to be the best way to avoid pregnancy. Molly first stopped taking them in 1978 and our first child, Adam, was born in 1979. Over the next ten years we tried various methods of pregnancy prevention. Everyone we had known in medical school, in residency, and later in rural practice in north Florida, seemed quite knowledgeable about various methods of birth control. They considered Rhythm at best silly and, for those women who should not get pregnant, a dangerous way to play at not getting pregnant. As for being faithful to the Church's teaching, we rebelliously questioned how a patriarchal group of celibate old men could foist their dangerous notions on poor, unsuspecting, women in need.

I had to overcome a few major intellectual hurdles on my way to NFP. While in college I became involved with various environmental protection groups on campus; a flattening of the population growth rate was preached as the key to solving the pollution problem and saving land from man's encroachment. I was a disciple of Paul Erlich, a writer who theorized the collapse of much of the world by starvation and the attendant environmental disaster from runaway overpopulation. A major tenet of the plan for the survival of society was the necessity of stopping the burgeoning numbers of ignorant, primitive peoples from procreating. The answer: America would provide developing nations with the pill, contraceptive foam, IUDs, sterilization, and in case of failure, abortion training. The replacement concept of population growth, i.e., one child per parent, maximum, made lots of sense to me. I heard women talk about: the burden of trying to raise children, when they could be better engaged in efforts to pull society from the brink; pregnancy robbing a woman of her otherwise unlimited future opportunity, while destroying her dreams for the future. I heard college-educated, seemingly intelligent and rational women speak of abortion in that rationale. I lived through the legalization of abortion in New Orleans in the early 1970s. I heard the intense verbal battles and rage in this conservative Catholic-dominated community. I bought into the idea that thoughtful women could reasonably decide to terminate their pregnancies. Abortion became an acceptable concept to me.

Then came medical school and my human embryology class. Dr. Ray Gasser boldly proclaimed that people were people from conception. Babies were shown to demonstrate reflexes as early as sixteen weeks gestation. I began to be swayed. In fact, I was never able to commit myself to personally promote abortion. Another life-changing event happened: our first child was conceived. We were pregnant! A marvelous feeling of creativity, love for my wife, dreams of the future with our now growing family, flooded over me. When Molly and I were dating and we talked about marriage, she said she wanted to have children with me. I was overwhelmed by her statement, that she cared enough about me, and projected far enough into our future to be able to make such a profound statement. The birth of our child had a profound effect on me; I changed. I could no longer be in favor of the right to abortion.

Still, I was well-indoctrinated in the issues of women's rights. I was the responsible doctor who makes healthcare available to society's most vulnerable. In my work environment, that meant the poor, black, barefoot, pregnant, grandmultiparous teenage patient at New Orleans Charity Hospital. Who could possibly deny contraception to these women? Most were single with multiple sexual partners. What other reasonable option existed? Sterilization frequently came to mind and was offered to nearly all the patients. I carried these ideas into my Family Practice residency in Tallahassee, Florida. As a fourth year fellow focused on obstetrics, I started two rural public health prenatal clinics and both supervised and performed hundreds of deliveries. I developed a very strong sense of commitment to the perceived needs of these women. The state was funneling many dollars into family planning services. I became expert at prescribing oral contraceptives, fitting diaphragms, and sterilizing both men and women. When they became available, I learned to insert Norplant and prescribe Depo-Provera injections. Ironically, I clung to a moratorium on IUD insertion, feeling strongly that the mechanism of action was abortifacient, a fact I'd retained from Dr. Gasser, the embryology professor from medical school years earlier. When we had our fourth child, I chose vasectomy sterilization as the best way to prevent further pregnancies — my gift to my wife, my pain as payment for hers endured with childbirth and child-rearing.

I entered the private practice of medicine in 1983, spent a year in New Orleans and then ventured into the woods of north Florida. After five years of private rural practice, I rejoined my residency program, this time as clinical faculty. While there, I was challenged during my contraceptive teachings and vasectomy instruction by two Catholic students. I had previously professed my Catholic beliefs and they had, in a marvelously open and non-confrontational way, expressed their decision to practice and prescribe NFP-only for their patients. One of those students, Dr. José Férnàndez, after finishing the residency training in Tallahassee, continued to pursue me for clarification of my ideas and to bring the Church's teaching to me. I remain grateful for this devout physician's continued efforts to bring this wonderful teaching of the Church to me. That was nearly nine years ago, and in the intervening years I have come to a very different place in presenting patients information about family planning. I have made the issue of family planning an opportunity for evangelization, at least to marvel with them at how they were put together so well by the Creator. I also decided I needed "to walk the walk." I had my vasectomy reversed, and my wife and I have been practicing NFP ourselves for a number of years now.

I have found new and very useful territory to explore about women's rights and opportunities: how the men in their lives could and should show respect for them, how men's control of their passions actually helps the relationship grow stronger, and how marriage can be strengthened by the practice of NFP. I have met many intelligent, strong-willed, independent thinking, rational women who have been able to grow careers outside the home, as well as many homemakers, who live the NFP commitment. I have come to see more clearly what the Church has been trying to say with the NFP message.

Concern for my patients first opened my heart and mind to NFP. I began to see a pattern where the contraceptive "help" I was prescribing to my healthy patients was not actually helping them, but potentially causing them harm. Physically, I was stunned by the many adverse reactions to hormonal contraceptives. The most startling was a case of a twenty-year-old woman who developed a 7 cm. benign liver tumor as a complication of the pill. The likelihood of encountering this complication is listed as 2/100,000. She required a major, risky, surgical procedure for cure — a procedure no local surgeon would even touch. She had to travel 200 miles to a liver transplant surgeon. That surgeon, on his follow-up note, described the lesion as a "classic birth control pill hepatic adenoma." Another patient, at the age of 27, had a heart attack, described by the cardiologist as caused by a combination of smoking and birth control pills. Three other patients had major dominant hemisphere strokes, all debilitating with one-sided weakness, unable to speak or care for themselves. A number of patients over the years have had clotting of the veins in their legs, several developing pulmonary emboli. In the early 1990s I was involved in the treatment of, or knew of, several previously healthy women in their early twenties who had taken the newest, very low-dose estrogen pill (two of the patients had taken the pill only a few months) when they developed complications. One of these three, a smoker, developed a headache and was found to have a small stroke on a brain CAT scan. Another developed showers of blood clots throughout her lungs. The third patient developed a blood clot which lodged in her lung and nearly killed her. All of these patients were hospitalized many days, requiring months of potent blood thinners for treatment. One of them will have to deal with life-long leg swelling. Many had much more severe residual effects. When I added these physical disasters, which were caused by hormonal contraceptive use, to the bleak social outcomes which result from unbridled sexual exploration, I searched to find other answers for my patients' needs in the arena of sexuality.

One of the most startling disease issues of our time has been the rise of the STD epidemic and the danger it poses, especially to women's health. The current epidemic is unprecedented in history, if only by the numbers of cases. For patients who are not in long-term monogamous relationships, I wanted them to be absolutely aware of the health risks posed by intercourse and other sexual activity when the condom is not used. My experience with teenagers who used a prescribed method of contraception other than the "mandatory" condom was that they would not use a condom even in high-risk situations. I concluded that my abstinence message was not getting across to these patients. Rather, the patients' use of birth control was encouraging a feeling of invincibility in sexual encounters. The best (or worst, perhaps!) were Depo-Provera and Norplant. These were seen as powerful shields, providing long-lasting protection, which the teenager did not even have to remember to take. As I looked at the side effect profile of these methods — patients who came in with "miscarriages" and Norplant in their arms, the huge weight gain of some patients, as well as the message of "safe sex" I was encouraging — I desired to quit these injectable forms of contraception as well. I began to give abstinence-based talks in the community instead of spending time promoting contraception.

Unfortunately, I was also caring for young women with HPV-related STDs that caused severe pre-cancerous changes of the cervix requiring surgical therapy. Condoms have been shown to be of no benefit in preventing the spread of HPV, weakening this foundation for the use of the condom. I tell folks that condom use is similar to wearing seat belts in a car speeding at 120 mph down a bad road — recommended perhaps, but with no guarantee of success.

Several patients whose tubes I'd tied came back to haunt me. They begged to know why I could not untie their tubes? They said they didn't know how much they'd want another baby later. Now they had found the man of their dreams and wanted to have a baby with him. Most of these patients are low-income women "I'd done a favor for." They could not begin to afford a tubal reversal and Medicaid certainly wasn't going to pay for it.

Finally, when the human embryo research project was winding its way through Congress in 1991-92, I found myself strongly defending the rights of the unborn to include protection from the date of conception on. When I found I could not under any circumstances allow even one abortion to take place by my hands, because of the contraception I had prescribed, I quit prescribing all forms of hormonal contraception including birth control pills.

When I went back into private practice in 1995, it was as an NFP-only doctor. I now am part of a clinic without walls, a large doctor group. I am also a provider physician for several HMO products. Patients enroll and pick a physician. Part of the services patients have come to expect from their doctor is contraception. I tell patients ahead of time that I do not prescribe contraception and that they will have to either change primary care providers or see one of the other providers for this service. Patients would have to make another appointment and pay the co-pay to that provider. I do not refer them to a contraceptive provider. Several plans allow abortions and sterilization. I have advised the plans that I will not refer for abortions. I try to discuss with patients the options to sterilization and disclose all risks and benefits of sterilization before they can see the urologist or gynecologist. Some patients have actually changed their minds when they understand the irreversible nature of this procedure.

I still struggle with the difficult dilemma of how to allow patients access to the services they feel they need without compromising my beliefs. This is a particular challenge for me here in this locale where not being on the HMO panel would be disastrous professionally. However, though abortions are a covered service under some plans, I have never, and will not ever, refer a patient for an abortion. My current practice patterns have helped me grow much closer to the Church, and I find that I am now much more open to the teachings of the Church on a broad range of issues.

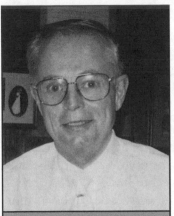

FOLLOWING THE HOLY SPIRIT

Dale L. Osterling, MD

Dr. Dale Osterling, a 1966 graduate of the University of Illinois College of Medicine, completed his residency in Obstetrics and Gynecology at the University of Colorado Medical Center. After a two-year tour with the U.S. Navy at the Naval Air Station Hospital in Jacksonville, Florida, Dr. Osterling settled into his present location in Inverness, Florida — where he has practiced medicine for 26 years. Since 1986 Dr. Osterling has limited his practice to gynecology.

Dale and his wife Jane center their lives around God and their large family. They have four biological daughters and two adopted sons. In 1975, following the sudden death of their best friends, they became guardians of four additional children. They are blessed with 14 grandchildren and feel fortunate to be able to see most of them frequently.

In March of 1998, after 26 years of practicing OB/GYN, I was led to discontinue prescribing contraception or performing sterilizations. Instead, I am recommending Natural Family Planning through the Couple to Couple League. This is how it happened.

Jane and I were married in 1962, two Catholics who met at a Methodist College, DePauw University in Greencastle, Indiana. Jane began working as an R.N. at Presbyterian-St. Luke's Hospital in Chicago as I began medical school at the University of Illinois. After one year of marriage and contracepting, we mutually decided to go to confession as we felt contraception was against God's will. We were told by the priest in the confessional that he couldn't tell us whether birth control was right or wrong and that we should, after prayerful consideration, do what we thought was the correct decision for us as individuals. We did decide to cease contracepting, but mainly because we were ready to begin a family. The experience did have a profound effect upon my professional actions later in life.

When our fourth daughter was born in early 1969, Jane went to confession because neither of us wanted any further children and contraception was definitely desired. In the confessional she was told she didn't need to have 100 children to prove her love for the church and he didn't have the authority to tell her whether contraception was right or wrong. An IUD was successfully used.

As contraception was a significant portion of OB/GYN training and practice, I prescribed oral contraceptives (OCs), inserted IUDs and performed sterilization with no sense of wrongdoing.

My OB/GYN residency at the University of Colorado in Denver from 1967-1970 exposed me to many abortions. Most were performed by saline instillation into the gravid uterus between 16-20 weeks of gestation. Colorado had a very liberal abortion law which antedated Roe vs. Wade. Frequently I was called upon to deliver the dead fetuses. I recalled how unpleasant it was dealing with the patients and their families as contrasted with obstetrical delivery experiences. I did not perform saline instillations but did perform one hysterotomy (for the medical indication of severe renal disease). I can still recall the metallic "tap tap" as the newborn 18-week fetus thrashed about after being placed in an empty coffee can in which it was sent to pathology.

As a result of the aforementioned experiences, I was determined to prevent abortions by prescribing OCs and inserting IUDs and performing sterilizations.

In the late 1980s, I ceased inserting IUDs. I viewed myself as pro-life and the pro-lifers stated that IUDs worked by causing abortion. I was even more uncomfortable with the economics of IUDs when they fell out or caused enough bleeding and cramps that removal was mandated. How much money do you refund under these circumstances? More for secular selfish reasons than being the right thing to do, I elected not to insert IUDs. I didn't enjoy dealing with dissatisfied customers.

The original birth control pills contained sufficient hormone to prevent ovulation 100% of the time. As the dosage was lowered to decrease the incidence of complications such as myocardial infarction, stroke, thrombophlebitis, and pulmonary embolus and death, it became apparent that ovulations began to occur. In 1996, when performing a tubal sterilization, I found multiple corpora albicantia, evidence of recent ovulations on the ovaries of women taking OCs. I was forced to confront the fact that at times OCs were interrupting pregnancy by preventing implantation of the conceptus. OCs were causing abortion.

Shortly thereafter, a surgical colleague, Tony Bescher, MD, inquired as to my feelings concerning contraceptives. I briefly went through what has heretofore been discussed. Tony and I conversed again the following week in the OR dressing room and I accepted a tape entitled "CONTRACEPTION: Why Not?" by Janet E. Smith, Ph.D. I listened to the tape with an initial detachment. Soon I found myself thinking "I'll have to show more support for Joyce and Steve Sablone," our local Couple to Couple League teaching couple. Later I found myself thinking, "I shouldn't be prescribing contraception. Not only is it wrong, but also very socially detrimental."

I had many long standing and treasured doctor-patient relationships that would be seriously affected if I followed through with action resulting from this revelation. I tried not to think about it.

Another discussion with Tony Bescher followed. We both attend weekly Eucharistic Adoration. Tony suggested praying for further guidance by the Holy Spirit and elimination of Satan's input into my thinking. At adoration I opened myself to Jesus and asked Him to enlighten me. I expected silence. Instead, within 5 seconds, I heard, "Read *Humanae Vitae*."

Humanae Vitae made so much sense. The act of love was given to married couples as a gift. Contraception defeated both the unitive and procreative intents of this gift. I knew I should no longer prescribe contraception or sterilization. I still delayed action.

The next week I carried the quarterly issue of *Sursum Corda*, still wrapped in cellophane, into Eucharistic Adoration. After prayers of thanksgiving and adoration, I opened myself to His inspiration. I immediately turned to an article entitled *The Return of the Catholic Doctor?* (Winter 1998). Multiple physicians told their story of how they had ceased prescribing contraception and how this decision has blessed them.

I then committed myself to cease providing contraceptive services and to promote natural family planning.

The Holy Spirit then helped me prepare a letter, which I sent to my patients to whom I prescribed contraception. This letter led to a story in the *St. Petersburg Times* which has given me encouragement as to the witness which is given when one acts upon his or her convictions. And Immaculata, Queen and Mother of the Church, is giving me new and exciting opportunities for being used for the coming of the kingdom of Jesus in the whole world.

GOD'S PLAN

Karen D. Poehailos, MD

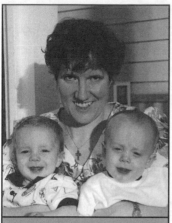

Dr. Poehailos graduated from the University of Virginia Medical School in 1989. She entered private practice after completing her residency in the University of Virginia's Family Medicine program, and is now balancing the practice of medicine with the demands of a young family. She and her family have recently relocated to Charlottesville, Virginia area, where she is currently working with First Med at Pantops, a group urgent medical center.

She is a member of Alpha Omega Alpha and was honored to receive the C. Richard Bowman Scholarship in 1988 — an award given to the UVa Senior medical student for clinical excellence and interpersonal skills in patient care. Karen and her husband Tony (Anthony W. Poehailos, III, MD — a child psychiatrist) are the parents

Natural Family Planning is often lauded as becoming a lifestyle, rather than just a method of regulating family size. This statement could not bear more truth, if what has happened in my family's life over the past two years has any bearing on others' experiences.

I have always considered myself pro-life ever since my Catholic high school days. Nothing about this changed during college, medical school, and family medicine residency. I never was asked to observe or participate in abortion, and learned all the gynecology required of a family physician, including prescribing oral contraceptives, fitting diaphragms, and even inserting IUDs. Unfortunately, I was unaware, from a pro-life aspect, of the implications of what I was doing, either not having learned it or taken the time to think about mechanisms of action.

of four boys: Anthony, age 5; Daniel, age 3; and 1-year-old twins, Patrick and Stephen.

I finished residency in 1992, and joined a group family practice in Annville, Pennsylvania, where I prescribed birth control pills, fit diaphragms, and, unfortunately, even once made an HMO referral for an abortion when I couldn't talk the patient out of it in the office. I thought I had no choice at the time, but later after discussing it with a priest in confession, I learned that under Pennsylvania laws I was under no obligation to make the referral, even if I was her PCP (Primary Care Physician). I never let that happen again.

My husband and I were introduced to NFP through our involvement in the Pre-Cana Program of the Harrisburg (Pennsylvania) Diocese, where we were a Lead Couple assisting in marriage preparation. My husband and I dutifully listened to the explanations, but as two physicians, we were rather skeptical of what sounded like the rhythm method, especially when the Catholic gynecologist who did my premarital exam dismissed it as impractical before discussing the alternatives. I think what finally persuaded us to give it a closer look was the discussion, given by our own pastor at one of the PreCana weekends, of the idea of giving God room to move in a marriage.

At the same time, I had been confronted by literature from the Priests for Life Organization that had been inserted in our parish bulletin regarding the abortifacient nature of the Pill, Norplant, and Depo-Provera. This in conjunction with a homily by our pastor about the lies propagated by Planned Parenthood made me start thinking, although initially, I confess I was thinking that our pastor had really overreached on that point and medically couldn't be right. Wouldn't I have learned that in seven years of medical school and family medicine residency training?

I hit the books on the matter to try to prove him wrong, but finally had to come to the conclusion that my pastor was absolutely correct, as was the Priests for Life brochure. The problem was, like any family physician (especially a female one), a good part of my practice involved gynecologic care. Many of these patients were on the Pill, which I justified in single patients by its potential to lower the unplanned pregnancy rate, as well as abortion demand. Fortunately, I had become convinced of the efficacy of NFP by this point; my husband and I had practiced it for several months, even during weaning our second child, and now saw how well I could interpret my body's signals. As a physician who always considered myself pro-life, could I continue to live with what I now knew to be a contradiction to that, or make the break from prescribing artificial contraceptives?

Fortunately, I lived in a diocese that is supportive of NFP. The diocesan NFP director was a great help to me, as were several doctors in the diocese and nearby areas who had made similar decisions and could offer practical advice. I met with my pastor to discuss all this, and he referred me to a diocesan priest who has his doctorate in medical ethics. After all the data gathering, and a lot of prayer, I decided to stop prescribing or referring for artificial contraception, and told my partners during Holy Week 1996. My office, at that time, was owned by a for-profit HMO, and I was concerned how they would accept my cutting off a large part of my gynecologic practice. By being organized enough to arrange for the care of my patients who wouldn't go along with my change of heart, I made it risk-free for them, as the patients could transfer within the practice and not affect their bottom line. The only risk would be my own, in productivity and patient satisfaction ratings. My coworkers, five physicians and two extenders, accepted my decision, though they did not agree with it.

I did lose some patients as a result, and had one father of a teenaged patient irately call to accuse me of patient abandonment, as she only wanted to see a female physician and not one of my male partners or the female extender. Largely, I saw my clientele switch in demographics to an older population, as the younger, sexually active patients migrated to my partners. My schedule was as full as ever, but more challenging, as I lost my younger, healthier patients.

God's ways are not necessarily our ways, a lesson rein-
forced for all of us since then. Five months after that, we
moved to Charlottesville, Virginia (in the diocese of Richmond), for professional reasons (not related to my becoming
NFP-only), and not without mixed emotions. On looking for
a job, I was able to find a practice where my not prescribing
artificial contraception would not be a problem. However,
there was really no NFP presence here, with the nearest
teaching couple being in Richmond (70 miles away). Now
only one year into practicing NFP myself, I found myself
looking into instructor classes. Again, to my rescue came the
NFP office in Harrisburg, where I was able to take an NFP instructor course on a long weekend visit.

Much of my time after that has been spent in NFP promotion with the local priests, some of the area physicians, and
the PreCana marriage preparation program. I had been invited to speak at a Pro-Life Symposium at my parish, as well
as deliver a grand rounds presentation at the University of
Virginia Family Medicine Department. The latter was particularly interesting, as I was going back to my old program. I
carefully researched the presentation, made handouts and
overheads, and was ready to shine. Unfortunately, attendance was fairly poor, and I'm not sure I convinced anyone
that NFP was viable, scientific, and worth their time. I was
frustrated afterwards when someone shared with me that
one of the flyers advertising my presentation had been al-
tered by someone with the line, "Ever wonder why Catholics
have so many kids?" I try to remember the admonition that
God only asks us to be faithful, not necessarily successful.

Thanksgiving weekend 1996 will always be one for my
husband and me to remember. On a visit back to Pennsylvania, I was going to teach my first NFP class to a couple from
my former parish. The day before I taught that class, we discovered that we were expecting a third child in early August
1997, a method-failure pregnancy. The scientist-side of me
was shocked (we followed all the rules) and how was I going
to ever be effective in promoting NFP here if I had this unplanned surprise? When I calmed down to more rational

thinking with the help of my husband and a few friends (and yes, did manage to teach that couple), I realized that God had a great lesson to teach me regarding NFP, that no doubt would be invaluable as I embarked on this adventure.

Over that past year, I became quite familiar with *Humanae Vitae* — intellectually. Yet, however much I professed to give God room to move in our marriage, I have to admit I really wanted it on my terms. My husband and I more fully came to realize to the depth of our souls that God had called this little one into being (NOT that NFP doesn't work). This is what *Humanae Vitae* was trying to say before it was so misinterpreted by the lay press — life is a gift from God and we need to let our lives be open to it. It was a good lesson to learn, especially when we discovered on an 18-week sonogram that I was carrying fraternal twins, our third and fourth sons!

Life has changed, to put it mildly — as I mother four sons ages 5, 3, and the 10 month old twins. I have largely set my family medicine career on hold, working one weekend a month at a University of Virginia Urgent Med. Center to keep my skills current. I have spent much of my "free" time in NFP promotion and teaching — about 20 couples in this past year — as well as working with Respect Life ministry and reviving a Eucharistic Adoration program at our parish. God clearly has had His hand in all this, as I am not sure how much time I would have been able to devote to these if I had continued my former position. I hope in a few years to be able to return to a part-time family medicine position so I can once again promote NFP in an office setting. As our dear former pastor in Pennsylvania (who continues as an advisor and friend for us since our move) put it: "You had a plan. God just has a better one." I pray to be open to see what He now wants from me — from us.

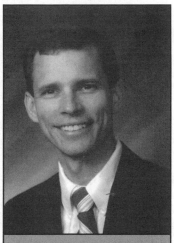

After graduating from the Michigan State University College of Osteopathic Medicine in 1984, Dr. Povich completed a residency in Family Practice. For the past three years he has been part of a group practice at the OSF Medical Group in Escanaba, Michigan. Mark and his wife Carol are busy parents of eight children ranging in ages from 19 to 2 — with #9 due this summer. The children's names are: Jordan, Jotham, Jocelyn, Joyanne, JoHannah, Josiah, Joseph and Joliette.

TRUTH AND CONSEQUENCES

Mark Povich, DO

My use of contraceptive agents early in my practice reflected the training I had received in medical school and family practice residency. I was bothered some by prescribing these to unmarried, often teenage, females who were involved in relationships that they eventually found to be hollow and self-destructive.

During my years in the Air Force, I frequently saw sexually transmitted diseases in the large unmarried population, but I reasoned that through the use of contraceptives I was at least preventing pregnancies that they would likely abort. My prescribing practices certainly never positively influenced behavior.

About this time I attended a Christian physician conference and was challenged to look at contraceptives as potentially abortifacient. Also reaffirmed was the concept that, within marriage, children are blessings from God and not burdens. Outside of marriage, pregnancy causes the woman or couple to need to make disconcerting choices, including possible abortion, adoption, or raising the child without the benefit of a stable marriage.

These uncomfortable choices are consequences of breaking God's commands. God uses consequences to get people's attention, to show them the error of their ways, and hopefully to motivate them to an obedient lifestyle. The removal of consequence enables these destructive behaviors to continue, and the prescribing of contraceptives makes the prescriber an enabler of immoral behavior by hindering God's consequences.

Even armed with this information, it still took a couple more years for me finally to decide to stop prescribing contraceptives. The initial battleground was in my heart, but now I am confident that I am in God's will. Subsequent battles revolved around the fear of others' responses to my decision, but I decided that it was more important that I had God's approval.

Fortunately, my colleagues accepted this departure from the status quo with a few polite questions. Some patients could not accept this change and transferred their care elsewhere.

As I continue in my walk as a Christian physician, I am seeing the need to become more bold and to lovingly challenge those engaged in immoral and destructive behavior. The more difficult groups to reach are Christians themselves, who have adopted many of the philosophies of the world. I am hopeful that my "Why I do not prescribe contraceptives" handout will cause all my patients to reflect on at least one aspect of how contraceptives may impact their lives, which may lead them into a deeper search for God's truth.

[Doctor Povich's handout "Why I do not prescribe
contraceptives" is in Appendix III.]

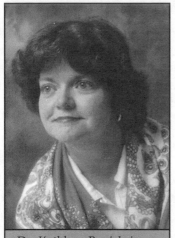

Dr. Kathleen Raviele is a board-certified gynecologist in solo practice in a suburb of Atlanta, Georgia. Dr. Raviele speaks regularly to RCIA programs, marriage preparation programs, pro-life groups and adult education programs. She also is the pro-life representative as well as an hourly coordinator for Perpetual Adoration in her parish.

Kathy lives with her husband Anthony and two teenage children, Angela and Nick, in Stone Mountain, Georgia.

A Gynecologist's Journey from Contraception to NFP

Kathleen Raviele, MD

As an obstetrician-gynecologist who has been on both sides of the fence in our culture of death, I can well appreciate the secular and economic pressures on Catholic physicians, today, to disregard the Church's teaching on legitimate means to space children. I, too, for 18 years thought there was no problem with performing sterilizations or prescribing contraception. After all, everyone around me did it, and patients expected it.

When Pope Paul VI issued his encyclical *Humanae Vitae* in 1968, I had just graduated from high school and already been accepted into a six-year BS/MD program. Listening to the feminist arguments and witnessing the examples around me which rejected the Church's teaching in this area, I also rejected it as being optional. I never thought to consult a priest before entering the field of obstetrics and gynecology.

Entering an internship-residency program at Case Western Reserve University in 1974, I cared for a predominately black, inner city patient population with a high out-of-wedlock pregnancy rate, so contraception and sterilization seemed the logical way to deal with this social problem.

My husband and I had been non-practicing Catholics for seven years when our first child was born in 1978. Her baptism by a priest at the Church of Our Lady of Peace started our journey back into the Catholic Church. When we moved to Atlanta, we immediately became friends with a Catholic family, comprising five children, and we went back to regular churchgoing.

For many years, first on the faculty at Emory University, and then in a busy group practice, I experienced no uncertainty or guilt about what I was doing on a daily basis. Occasionally, I would wonder if I was doing any good handing out birth control pills to a sixteen-year-old, thinking it would prevent her from having an abortion, only to see her get a STD or get pregnant and have the abortion anyway. I was also amazed to see so many marriages breaking up after one spouse had been sterilized.

Then in 1989, my husband's brother Frank became terminally ill. We brought him to our home for the last three months of his life, and it proved to be a major turning point for me. Out of the Church for his entire adult life, he was reconciled with God through a priest we knew well. The priest came every Saturday for thirteen weeks to hear Frank's confession and give him Holy Communion; the priest anointed him the day before he died. Frank's illness and death made me start thinking about eternity.

The following year, my children brought home a newsletter from their parochial school that had a paragraph stating that the Blessed Mother had been allegedly appearing to six young people in Medjugorje, Yugoslavia, since 1981, and that each Thursday we should read Matthew 6:24-34. Taking our never-opened Bible out of the drawer, I read in the passages that we cannot serve two masters, God and money. I thought to myself that I didn't worship money.

Six months later, I read Wayne Weible's book, *Medjugorje: the Message*, and had a sudden blinding conversion experience as a door that had been opened only a crack flew wide open, and a blinding light shone into my heart. I believed everything! My children and I started doing what Our Lady was asking. We prayed the Rosary together each day, read out of the Bible, started going to confession monthly, fasted on Wednesday and Friday, prayed for peace, and I started going to Mass on Saturday and my day off.

Although I thought I was doing all these acts of piety for others, I found myself becoming acutely aware of things I needed to change in my life. My relationship with my children, which was already good, became even closer because of praying together. I talked with two priests about my job, but I was told that these are difficult times and just to do my best.

Feeling an overwhelming desire to visit Medjugorje, I took my children, ages 10 and 12, and did so in June of 1991. I felt part of the reason I needed to go was to find something out, but I didn't expect it to be about my career. At the time we were there, there were about 150,000 people from all over the world. Lines for confession were long, but after four days, I felt I needed to speak with the Glenmary priest who was with our group. After I explained to him what I did in my job, he told me I needed to stop what I was doing. He said the Church had been unwavering in this teaching since the time of Christ and that it was in Scripture and in the tradition of the Church. He told me how contraception had led to teenage promiscuity, abortion, divorce, widespread homosexual activity, pedophilia, and that it broke all ten of God's commandments. He told me I needed to leave my practice and then I would have more time for my family.

I was shocked to hear all these things. I did not understand why contraception was wrong, but as I looked into his eyes and then at the beautiful fields, mountains and blue sky that day, I knew that was why Our Lady had called me there. She wanted me to listen to Her Son without any distractions — she wanted me to hear the truth.

Returning to the real world, I thought I could stay where I was and just stop prescribing contraception and doing sterilizations. However, it soon became evident that this was not possible, and I left a prosperous practice of five physicians, where I was a senior partner, to start a solo gynecology practice. With no Catholic hospitals in the city doing obstetrics, cross coverage with other OB/GYNs would have been difficult because of the large number of tubal ligations done at the time of cesarean section.

Learning about natural family planning was not easy. There were few teachers in my diocese. I trained first to be a symptothermal teacher because there were three symptothermal programs being taught. Then in 1996, I went through the Medical Consultant program at the Pope Paul VI Institute. There I learned about all the medical applications of NFP in infertility, ovarian cysts, and premenstrual syndrome, all in keeping with the teachings of the Church. Now at the completion of the Practitioner program, teaching the Creighton Ovulation Method has been an awesome experience as I have gotten to know couples and helped them with their struggles to remain chaste before marriage, shared with them their sorrow and stress over being infertile, and marveled at their growth in trust and mutual respect for each other as they learn the method. What an incredible treasure the Church has in modern natural family planning.

At the end of each workday, I thank God for showering His great mercy upon me and healing my blindness. I ask that He heal other physicians' blindness, too, because there are many well-intentioned doctors who would do what is right if they learned the truth and if they had the faith to accept it. It is not a coincidence that since 1990, several OB/GYNs, like me, have had a change of heart. In every case, a spiritual renewal in their life coincided with the change. Those of us who have made the change are ready and willing to support the physicians who wonder if it can be done.

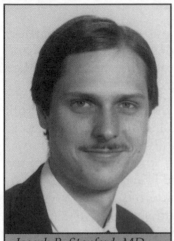

Joseph B. Stanford, MD, CNFPMC, is assistant professor in the Department of Family and Preventive Medicine at the University of Utah School of Medicine in Salt Lake City. He obtained his M.D. degree from the University of Minnesota, and completed his family practice specialty training at the University of Missouri-Columbia. He also received a Master's Degree in Public Health from the University of Missouri-Columbia.

Dr. Stanford is active in research in human fertility and Natural Family Planning. He has also been involved in the American Academy of Natural Family Planning (AANFP) and, as of July 1998, is serving as President of that Organization. Joe and his wife Kathleen have five sons — Matthew, Jesse, Hyrum, Caleb and Thomas.

MY PERSONAL AND PROFESSIONAL JOURNEY WITH REGARD TO MORAL ISSUES IN HUMAN PROCREATION

Joseph B. Stanford, MD, MSPH

When I was completing my baccalaureate in Mankato, Minnesota, in 1984, I had no idea that 14 years later, as an academic family physician, I would be fully committed to promoting an understanding of human sexuality and procreation which is radically at odds with the prevailing views and practices of our contemporary culture. But through those 14 years, I have found that one of the most meaningful causes of truth to which I give my personal and professional effort is striving to promote understanding of truths about the miracle of human procreation. In sketching my life's journey in relation to these issues, I would hope to help others, particularly health professionals, to consider their own values and examine their conscience with regard to the vital choices they make when dealing with human procreation.

From my earliest age, I learned from my parents, by both example and precept, the inestimable value of the virtue of chastity. Though I did not always fully appreciate its importance in my younger years, this principle has been one of the guiding lights of my life, a rock solid foundation for my marriage, and the background that made me able to recognize and understand truths about human sexuality as I encountered them in my life. Thus I was ready to listen when I first heard about natural family planning during my first year of marriage, which was also my first year of medical school.

After returning from two years of missionary service for the Church of Jesus Christ of Latter-day Saints, I had determined to complete a Ph.D. in biochemistry and do research related to human nutrition, but was persuaded by an interview with my stake president (ecclesiastical leader) to enter medicine as my profession. In medical school, I found that my interest in both the physical and spiritual aspects of health translated into a desire to have a holistic view of the entire person and family, and so I pursued a career in family medicine.

During my first semester of medical school, there was a noon lecture series on "alternative medicine" topics organized by medical students to cover items not addressed in our medical school curriculum (such as acupuncture, hypnosis, etc.). My wife Kathleen joined me for a brown bag lunch at many of these lectures, since she was also attending the University of Minnesota to complete her degree in chemistry. One of the lectures that we attended together was on natural family planning, and was given by Dr. Dennis O'Hare from Twin Cities NFP, and Jim and Mary Glover from the Couple to Couple League (CCL). Immediately after the lecture, we both said to each other that this is exactly what we wanted in our marriage. We attended CCL classes in St. Paul, taught by

Mike and Mary Gaida. We felt a little bit awkward with some of the Catholic references, but we really enjoyed what we learned, for the first time, about our fertility as a married couple. We continued our use of the sympto-thermal method as taught by CCL for the next five years, and through the conceptions and births of our first two sons. In addition to NFP, things we learned from CCL about breastfeeding (including the concept of ecological and extended breastfeeding) and parenting (including the ideas of the family bed) have been of great benefit in our family life.

In our pharmacology class during the second year in medical school, we were taught that the primary mechanism of hormonal contraception was the alteration of the endometrium to not allow implantation of the conceptus. (I have since come to realize that this was actually overstated, but nevertheless it got me thinking at the time.) A small group of us in the medical school class decided that because of this, we would not prescribe hormonal contraceptives. Those that made this commitment included a Catholic, a Baptist, (both women), and myself. I don't know for sure about my classmates, but I have since stuck with that decision throughout my training and practice. This has opened the way for me to grow and learn in other ways that would not otherwise have been possible, and it has also allowed me to give much to my patients that otherwise I might never have been able to offer.

My wife and I felt strongly enough about the value of NFP that early on, we applied to be a teaching couple for CCL. At the time, we were rejected, which was a big disappointment. In the final analysis, this was because, at that time, I had not yet decided that I would not prescribe barrier methods of contraception in my future medical practice. For the next few years, I wrestled with the issues of contraceptives that were not potentially abortifacient, as well as with the issue of sterilization. I did not resolve these issues until the middle of my residency. During this time, I counseled with my bishop in my Church, and at his advice also wrote a letter to a prominent authority of the Church. He wrote back to me and said that I should seek the inspiration of the Lord in making my decisions about how to practice medicine, and that if I did so in sincerity, the Holy Ghost would guide me to make the right decisions. He suggested that I live my life with the constant realization that I would one day give account to the Lord Jesus Christ for my choices, including my decisions in the practice of medicine. I have since lived by this, and have been richly blessed for it.

Another decision that I made during my medical training stands out in my mind. One of the required courses of our medical school was a weekend "human sexuality attitude reassessment" seminar. The course included several hours of hard-core pornographic films, used to "broaden" students' perspectives on human sexuality. Buried in the course syllabus was the possibility of opting out of that weekend seminar by writing a paper on my personal attitudes on human sexuality and how they would affect the care that I would give patients who had attitudes different from mine. I joined three or four of my classmates (out of our class of 120) in writing a paper instead of attending the weekend seminar. That paper, in and of itself, was a blessing in helping me clarify my thoughts on the sacredness of human sexuality.

When it came time to interview for a residency in my chosen field of family medicine, I did not talk about my decision not to prescribe hormonal contraception (or put in IUDs) until my second residency interview, when a perceptive (and supportive) residency director questioned me about my feelings in this regard. He indicated that he felt that it was important for me to share my stance with the programs that I interviewed at, and so I did for all of the rest of my interviews. One of the residency programs told me that they could not accept me if I did not prescribe birth control pills, but the rest of the programs indicated willingness to respect my stance and work with me, even if they found this an odd viewpoint. (I know from many colleagues and friends that OB-GYN programs in general are much less accommodating of individuals who hold such views. It is all but impossible for an OB-GYN resident to get through a program without prescribing hormonal contraceptives.) One family medicine program, in particular, indicated that they had a previous resident with similar viewpoints whom they had respected highly and with whom they had been able to work out a positive approach. This was the program that I ranked first (for many reasons not limited to this issue) and matched in — the University of Missouri-Columbia.

Once I started residency, I was not sure at first how to handle some of the issues that were thrown at me, such as phone calls for birth control refills while I was on call, use of birth control pills for non-contraceptive purposes, and many others. I decided to look up the former resident who had blazed the trail for me in the residency. I tracked down Michael Dixon in Kansas City, and drove there one weekend, where I had a chance to talk with him until the very late hours of one night. Michael was there for me precisely when I needed him and had a great impact on my life. I consider him a good friend, even though I have seen him less than a dozen times since then. If I had not met him, I may well have not persisted in my decision, faced with countless daily "practical" dilemmas on this issue. In that late night talk, he gave me three things, each of which was invaluable in its own right: 1) practical tips for negotiating residency training in a way that could respect the choices of both patients and colleagues while still being true to my own choice of conscience not to prescribe hormonal contraception; 2) perspectives and issues that helped me begin to consider that I might wish to choose not to prescribe any artificial contraception, not just abortifacients; and 3) that there are expansive options for gynecologic health based on approaches that respect and restore (rather than suppress) natural fertility. With regard to the latter, Michael introduced me for the first time to the medical research and insights of the Creighton Model Ovulation Method, to the advanced medical training in NFP available through the Pope Paul VI Institute for the Study of Human Reproduction, and to the American Academy of Natural Family Planning, which was to become an important part of my life. Sometime after this, my wife and I began using the

Creighton Model Ovulation Method, which we have used through the conceptions and births of our third, fourth, and fifth sons. Michael has since become one of the handful of physicians in the country who successfully completed residency training in obstetrics and gynecology while not prescribing contraceptives or performing sterilization. (There are many more obstetrician-gynecologists who have decided not to do so sometime after having completed their training.)

I am forever grateful for Michael being there at the right time and place to support my journey. I have tried to pass on the favor whenever I could. During the time that I was a family medicine resident, a chief resident, and subsequently a fellow at the University of Missouri-Columbia, I helped four other residents make and stick with similar choices not to prescribe forms of contraception that went against their conscience. Two of these were Catholic and two were Protestants. I helped to form an official residency policy on the issue, which is in place at that residency to this day. During residency, I also gave my first few talks to medical audiences about NFP. At this time, long-distance contact with obstetrician-gynecologist and NFP pioneer Hanna Klaus, MD provided crucial support to me in these steps.

During my residency, I had virtually no requests to fit diaphragms. I also did not seek to learn to do tubal ligations or vasectomies (like some of my family practice colleagues do) because of statements by LDS Church leaders strongly discouraging these procedures. With regard to sterilization, I also recognized that fertility is a part of health, not a disease, and so there is something fundamentally contradictory about doing a surgery to remove a healthy and fundamental function of the body. Over time and experience with patients, I began to feel that any form of contraception had its unintended detrimental effects on the marital (or non-marital) relationship, whether recognized or not. Based on my understanding that sexuality and fertility are linked at the most fundamental level both physically and spiritually, I began to see more and more clearly what can unfortunately happen when man tries to undo this link that is so deeply a part of nature in general, and of the marital relationship in particular. The sexual union in marriage is meant to be a complete giving of each spouse to the other, and when fertility (or potential fertility) is deliberately excluded from that giving, I am convinced that something valuable is lost. I have observed that a husband can come to see his wife as an object of sexual pleasure, who should always be available for gratification. This is more likely, given that the dominant perspective on sexuality in our society is that of unlimited sexual titillation and gratification, which is (theoretically) freed from any consideration of pregnancy. Especially, methods such as sterilization and hormonal contraceptives feed into this prevalent and very distorted male perspective, which is also adopted by many women. Couples can also easily lose sight of why they have made a decision to avoid pregnancy and not discuss the issue for months or years, when they would be better off considering the issue on an ongoing basis.

At the same time, I am persuaded, both by research and direct experience with patients, that those couples who do have a serious consideration to avoid pregnancy can reliably do so by using NFP. The periodic abstinence of NFP can be challenging, even at times very difficult, but it strengthens marriages as each spouse puts the needs of each other and their marriage ahead of their own needs. There is also a "courtship/honeymoon" effect that can help develop non-genital aspects of the relationship, and increase the appreciation and enjoyment of the sexual union when it happens. I have known couples in my practice using artificial contraception who routinely have daily intercourse, but these couples do not have nearly as satisfying of a "sex life" as those couples I see who use NFP. Simply put, I believe that NFP enhances marriages in a way that the use of artificial contraception does not. There are also medical side effects of greater or lesser nature with every contraceptive. All of these considerations brought me to the point that I simply could not participate in prescribing something that I feel is ultimately detrimental to marriage and to the health of the spouses. All this was confirmed for me by the decision I made midway through my residency that I could not in conscience prescribe contraceptives of any sort (whether or not they are abortifacient) for my patients.

I find that the following benefits come to those couples who use NFP: 1) they come to a deeper appreciation of fertility as a gift from God, rather than a biological phenomenon to be manipulated or a curse to be avoided; 2) they are usually able to consciously and rapidly achieve pregnancy when they choose to ("surprise" pregnancies are rare for NFP users); 3) they consider their choices about their fertility on an ongoing basis; 4) in their relationship, each spouse sends to the other the implicit and powerful message: "I accept all of you, including your fertility"; 5) they learn to assume and exercise joint responsibility for decisions about their fertility; and 6) they learn that times of abstinence from genital contact can strengthen their relationship. I have also observed that a message from a physician that says "I cannot in conscience prescribe contraceptives, but I can fully recommend NFP without reservations" carries much more weight in helping patients really consider the idea of using NFP than "I think NFP is the best and healthiest method, but whatever you choose I will be happy to prescribe for you." Don't misunderstand me here: I have not taken my own stand simply to put across a more potent message to patients about NFP; this is simply my observation of what has happened since I have made my stand (and in observing other physicians who have or have not done so).

Most people who start to use NFP do not do so because they expect to experience the benefits to their relationship and spirituality that I have just described. Rather, my research suggests that a majority are interested primarily for the health benefits (the absence of medical side effects and the insight into the normal functioning of the body). Others begin use of NFP because of a prior religious commitment to this form of family planning. Regardless of the reason for beginning use of NFP, most research has shown that relatively high proportions of users continue use of it, compared to other family planning methods. And after some months of use, most users will tell you that they have noticed some of the benefits to their relationships that I described earlier.

All of this does not mean that I presume in any way to judge others (particularly not my patients) when they choose to use contraceptives. Their choices about their reproductive potential are between themselves and God, if/when they recognize God, and it is their right and responsibility to determine for themselves what they will do about their fertility. I am most willing to talk about all of the family planning options with all my patients, freely acknowledging what my own perspective and bias is. I do strive to be balanced in discussing my medical assessments for various contraceptive methods. It is not my purpose to attack contraception. Further, it is simply not appropriate to overstate medical side effects of any contraceptive, or to understate its effectiveness to avoid pregnancy for the purposes of persuasion. Such tactics are not fully honest if consciously employed, and in any case will usually backfire. In the process of discussions with patients on these issues, I clearly let them know what I can and cannot do within my own conscience, and that they will need to go elsewhere if they choose an option that I cannot participate in. My experience has been that almost all my patients are very understanding of this. Almost all my patients who do end up choosing to use prescription contraception have returned to me for the rest of their medical care. I have found that approximately one-fourth of my patients who did not previously use NFP choose to do so after having such a discussion with me. (On the other hand, many of my patients sought me out to be their physician because of their knowledge that I am one of a very few physicians who will support their prior choice to use NFP.)

I also do not mean to imply in any way that couples who use contraception will necessarily have bad marriages or family problems. I know many wonderful couples who are very open to life and completely committed to their families and yet also use contraceptives. Very many of them have very successful families. Yet, I remain convinced that most if not all of these couples would switch to NFP if they had the opportunity to really understand it and the further blessings that they would derive from using it. Many people who use contraceptives would never consider abortion for a "surprise pregnancy", but it is a quite different story when you look at those who have developed contraceptives and promoted them on political and social levels to their current level of acceptance in our society (and such widespread acceptance is still only a few decades old). I think that it is highly instructive that, almost without exception, those who support and fund the development and dissemination of contraceptives come from a perspective that sees abortion as an essential and fundamental backup to "contraceptive failure" so that women can be totally "freed" from the biology of their fertility, and from a perspective that lists population control, even if by coercive methods, as one of the most important issues of our time.

The issues are similar with regard to those who prescribe contraceptives. In my opinion, there are far too many providers who do not hesitate to push their values of limiting family size on their patients. For example, one common form of this is to ask a woman going to a C-section if she wants to take advantage of the surgery to get her tubes tied. Her decision at that time, especially after having gone through a difficult pregnancy, will not necessarily reflect the decision she might make after reflection months later. Yet there are many providers who highly value human life and have a Christian (or otherwise God-centered) perspective on the value of family life, who still prescribe contraceptives or do sterilizations. Again, I do not in any way presume to judge them for their decisions. Those decisions are between each of them and God. But I have a moral responsibility to judge for myself my own actions in the practice of medicine and seek inspiration from the Lord for doing so. When I get to the judgment bar of Christ, I cannot say, "Well, I just did what all of my colleagues did, what was the medical standard of care." In addition to forming my own moral conscience by the inspiration of the Holy Spirit, I also must share what I have found with anyone who is ready to hear so they can consider these issues for themselves and seek the Lord's guidance in their lives. It seems likely to me that relatively few Christian providers have really done so. Because I respect the moral agency of other providers, I have found that many faculty in my residency and most colleagues in my practice have been very supportive of my right to practice according to my conscience, even those that have fundamentally and strongly disagreed with me.

This is not to say that I have been totally free of misunderstanding or discrimination due to my stand on these issues. At the time that I finished my fellowship and interviewed for positions in academic medicine, I was very up front in my discussion of these issues during my job interviews. I found that one faculty member at a state university was very concerned about my pro-life orientation, which may have cost me an offer at that institution. Curiously, the one place where I met with vehement antagonism because I did not prescribe contraceptives was at a Catholic medical school where I interviewed. I had other options open to me, however, and I have ended up at the University of Utah in Salt Lake City, where I have a thriving practice and research program.

My research interests were supported in medical school by a research advisor. In addition, I had met with Konald Prem, MD, a faculty gynecologist who encouraged my desire to do research in NFP. During residency, I was able to pursue these interests with support from faculty and collaborators sympathetic to NFP, including Janis Lemaire, FNP. As I pursued further research training during a fellowship, I continued to focus most of my research efforts in NFP and related areas.

While yet in residency, I closed one loop in my life by contacting Dennis O'Hare, who was serving as Chairman of the Science and Research Committee of the American Academy of Natural Family Planning. I submitted some of my research for presentation at the annual meeting of the American Academy of Natural Family Planning (AANFP), which was accepted. There I began many wonderful associations and friendships which have blessed my life to this day. When

I had previously served as an LDS missionary in southern Germany, I had met countless Christmas/Easter Catholics whose commitment to their religion seemed almost entirely social. The Catholics I met at the AANFP, like those I had met previously in our associations with the Couple to Couple League, are of an entirely different sort. These are wonderfully committed people whose faith profoundly informs their entire life and service. I would like to make particular mention of my friendship with Thomas W. Hilgers, MD, which started at that meeting. In him I found not only a research colleague, but a man of the deepest integrity and commitment to life and to God. I count him as perhaps my most significant mentor in medicine, particularly with regard to integrating spirituality with medicine, and faith with exacting scientific inquiry. Soon after that first meeting, I completed the Medical Consultant Training Course In Natural Family Planning run by Dr. Hilgers at the Pope Paul VI Institute for the Study of Human Reproduction in Omaha, Nebraska. I have since attended the annual meeting of the AANFP every year. It is a wonderful meeting where deep faith and rigorous science meet and dialogue in the service of understanding and teaching the wonderful truths about the miracle of human fertility. The members of the AANFP are among my closest friends. I have served for a number of years as Chairman of the Science and Research Committee, and am currently serving as president-elect. The fact that I am one of a very few non-Catholic members of that organization has not hindered my deep friendship and common purpose with these wonderful people on issues that are of fundamental, if largely unrecognized, importance to all of humanity. I have also had the opportunity for a number of years to serve as faculty for training programs for health professionals in NFP, including the annual Medical Consultant Training Course at the Pope Paul VI Institute, where increasing numbers of physicians (over a dozen each year) are being trained in a perspective on reproductive medicine which is fully respectful of life and fertility.

My Catholic friends often ask me what the LDS Church stance is on contraception. There are very few recent statements from LDS Church authorities explicitly on the subject of contraception, but statements by Church leaders have made very clear the following relevant doctrinal points:

1. Human life is sacred from the moment of conception.
2. Chastity is of central importance both outside and inside marriage.
3. Marriage is a cornerstone of God's plan for humankind.
4. There is a divinely mandated and inseparable link between sexuality and procreation.
5. The body is a sacred gift from God and a central part of the purpose for our earthly life.
6. The body is the temple for the Holy Spirit.
7. It is vitally important that we do nothing that would harm or injure the health or normal function of the body.
8. In this mortal life we need to search out, learn, and live by the laws that govern our earthly lives.
9. The first commandment given to married couples to multiply and replenish the earth is still valid.
10. Children are "an heritage of the Lord," the Lord's blessings to a married couple.
11. Family life is where the greatest blessings of life are found.
12. Each husband must be respectful of his wife's health and well-being.
13. Parents must carefully seek divine inspiration to plan for and care for their families.
14. Self-control and mutual respect are vitally important components of the marriage relationship.

A recent proclamation on the family by the First Presidency and Council of the Twelve Apostles of the Church states, "The first commandment that God gave to Adam and Eve pertained to their potential for parenthood as husband and wife. We declare that God's commandment for His children to multiply and replenish the earth remains in force. We further declare that God has commanded that the sacred powers of procreation are to be employed only between man and woman, lawfully wedded as husband and wife. We declare the means by which mortal life is created to be divinely appointed. We affirm the sanctity of life and of its importance in God's eternal plan." To me, all of these doctrines in their fullness completely support the appropriateness of using NFP within marriage, both in theory and in practice. It is possible for a couple to use NFP in an inappropriate way to selfishly limit their family, but in my opinion, this is much less likely to happen with NFP than it is with the use of artificial methods of contraception.

Of course, I have become quite familiar with Catholic perspectives (as well as dissent among Catholics) on these issues. I have taken the opportunity to read and reread *Humanae Vitae*, the 1968 encyclical of Pope Paul VI. Although there are some theological points in it with which I disagree, I find myself in complete agreement with the fundamental vision of human sexuality and family life, which is beautifully set forth. I believe that the insights of that encyclical could only have come from divine inspiration. Similarly, though I cannot agree with every detailed point of Pope John Paul II's *Evangelium Vitae*, I find the clarity of the vision on the complete understanding of the battle between the culture of life and the culture of death breathtakingly illuminative. It has also been my great privilege to meet Pope John Paul II in Rome in November 1994, during a meeting held by the Pontifical Academy of Sciences on NFP research.

As a medical school faculty member, research related to NFP has become the main basis of my research funding. I have presented on NFP and NFP-related research at dozens of medical meetings. Attendance at my sessions is almost always sparse, and often a large share of the audience leaves immediately prior to my presentation. Apparently, they know everything they want to know on the topic. But there are always a few who listen, which makes it worthwhile. There is essentially no support for NFP among pharmaceutical companies, which makes for a hard road in getting the message out to health professionals. There are many old myths to overcome related to the calendar rhythm method (myths which are not even accurate with regard to that outdated method of NFP). In this regard, a change of terms may prove helpful in the near future, since "natural family planning" has come to be associated with pejorative connotations both among health professionals and among the public.

Among health professionals, there are various levels of commitment to NFP. A level that I hope to see the majority of health professionals in the United States come to in my lifetime, notwithstanding all forces to the contrary, is the acceptance and promotion of NFP as an option which should be available to all women and couples. (Currently the number of NFP teachers in the U.S. is pitifully small and distributed such that many people in the population do not have access to quality instruction in NFP.) Even those health professionals who are committed to contraception and who may countenance abortion have the potential to come to this level of support given adequate data on NFP effectiveness, although those who come from a perspective of population control will always remain suspicious of NFP because it seemingly makes it too easy for a couple to get pregnant without what they would consider adequate motivation to do so. There are other health professionals who strongly promote the many health benefits of NFP, while still maintaining a perspective that sees NFP as essentially one of many methods of contraception, whatever its advantages might be. Others, like myself, come sooner or later to realize that NFP differs fundamentally from contraception in that it cooperates with the divine gift of fertility, rather than seeking to suppress or destroy it, and that cooperating with the divine gift of fertility brings spiritual blessings as well as medical benefits. I will gladly work with people from each of these perspectives on all areas of common ground to see that this incredible and still largely undiscovered gift of knowledge from the Creator reaches His children throughout the world.

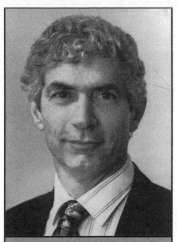

*Dr. William Toffler, a 1976
graduate of the Medical College
of Virginia, is currently a
professor and the Director of
the Education Section of the
Department of Family
Medicine at Oregon Health
Sciences University.*

*Dr. Toffler continues to be
actively committed to defending
the long-standing prohibition against doing harm and
to directly opposing physi-
cian-assisted suicide (PAS)
and active euthanasia. He is
frequently invited to speak
about PAS and other related
ethical issues at both
regional and national
conferences.*

*Dr. Toffler is co-founder
and National Director of
Physicians for Compassionate Care Education Foundation (PCC), a non-profit
organization which promotes
compassionate care for*

COMPROMISE, CONSISTENCY AND CHRISTIANITY ONE PHYSICIAN'S JOURNEY TOWARD THE TRUTH

William Toffler, MD

While I was raised a Catholic and had never openly rejected my Christian heritage, I was also clearly a product of our American culture. In our diverse society, I was taught to avoid judgments and that I had no right to assert my own moral views on others. On the other hand, as a Christian I knew that the taking of innocent life was unacceptable. Specifically, I knew that abortion was wrong.

Yet as a medical student in the early '70s, I hadn't really thought much about how my own beliefs would interface with actual medical practice. As such, I wasn't really prepared for the dilemma that I would face in my 3rd year *severely-ill patients without sanctioning or assisting their suicide. PCC, having begun in Oregon, has more than 1300 members and is growing rapidly with physician members throughout the country.*

Bill and his wife Marlene are the parents of seven children (ages 6-20) who, as he says, "handily keep them from wondering what to do with their free time."

while on an Obstetrics rotation. One day on that rotation, my classmate Marian (not her real name) and I were assigned to the East Hospital, where indigents received care. Our resident had been assigned the task of performing saline abortions and several women in their second trimester lay on gurneys lined up like airplanes taxiing on a runway before takeoff. Marian and I watched the resident as neither of us had ever previously witnessed the procedure.

It seemed pretty simple. First cleanse the skin on the mother's abdomen with betadine. Insert a long needle into the uterus and withdraw amniotic fluid. Then inject the contents of two syringes, each filled with a large volume of salt solution, into the fluid sac surrounding the baby. The procedure was completed by withdrawing the needle. The mother could now return to the floor (where labor would subsequently ensue and the dead baby would be passed vaginally).

The whole process took less than three minutes. I stood in silence as the mother was taken away by an attendant. My classmate Marian, who was always eager to learn new procedures, was more animated. She asked the resident, "Can I do one?" The resident paused momentarily, then nodded affirmation. Marian cautiously repeated the simple steps under the watchful eyes of the resident. Everything went smoothly. After Marian was done, she seemed even more energized. She was smiling and, after a brief moment, Marian turned to me. "Bill, why don't you do one?"

The question took me off-guard. While I knew where I stood personally, I didn't want to appear judgmental. After all, wasn't the woman going to have the abortion anyway? What difference would it make who actually did the procedure? What would they think if I declined? Without further delay, I responded, "Sure, why not?" Over the next few minutes, I completed the same steps as readily as had the resident and my classmate. I didn't think much about what I had done at the time. I don't remember even talking about it. If I had any feelings then, I must have pretty well stuffed them. No one else seemed bothered and thus why would I? I simply blended in. As confused as I was in my thinking about abortion at the time, I was even more confused about contraception.

Despite my Catholic roots, I was blind to any connection between artificial birth control and abortion. If I may have had a vague sense that the church frowned on birth control, I thought it was really more a matter of individual conscience, not a serious problem. In fact, shortly after Marlene and I married, she and I both liked the idea of an intrauterine device (IUD). It seemed like a carefree approach for both of us and yet the responsible way to act. I thought we should avoid children until I was out of medical school when I judged we could better afford being parents. When her request to have the IUD placed was refused by her doctor because of his concerns about such devices in women who hadn't yet had a baby, I was taken aback — even a bit angry. After all, what right did he have to impose his views or beliefs if Marlene and I were both willing to accept the risks? While Marlene and I were perturbed, we didn't persist with our request nor did we seek another opinion or care provider.

I didn't realize it at the time, but this incident was to serve as an important lesson that I now share with students, residents and practicing colleagues. Clearly, physicians have a profound impact on their patients. Their willingness (or unwillingness) to share their values greatly influences decisions made by patients. When the IUD was subsequently taken off the market because of the significant morbidity (and even mortality) to thousands of women, I was thankful that her physician had not simply acted like "a vending machine." But that's another story and I don't want to get ahead of myself.

I had no difficulty learning to prescribe the pill and to insert IUDs. In fact, in my second year of residency, I regularly staffed a family planning clinic for the County Health Department. I avoided imposing my judgment and even put IUDs in teens who had never been pregnant— as long as they knew the risks. Prescribing pills, even in older women who smoked, wasn't a problem for me either. Again, I just explained the risks. In fact, I prided myself on my openness to all options. Obviously, at that time in my residency I didn't appreciate the wisdom of my wife's doctor. Instead, I let my patients make some bad choices in a value-neutral climate.

In practice, contraception was a big part of what I did. I was good at procedures and learned to deftly perform vasectomies. I inserted hundreds of IUDs. One of my first questions before discharging a new mother after her delivery was "What kind of contraceptive do you want?" If a tubal ligation was desired, I assisted. If a mother wanted an abortion, I would try to offer other options, even encourage her to adopt or connect her with helping agencies such as Crisis Pregnancy or Birthright. Yet, if she persisted with her desire for termination, I would also help her make the connection with an abortionist. I followed the logic that I had grasped and internalized in that awkward moment in my third year of medical school— "Well, she is going to do it anyway and I may as well help."

Looking back, I was a regular practitioner of situational ethics. I made compromises that, while understandable, were nonetheless wrong. Still, I was comfortable with myself and my practice. Attitudinal change would not come quickly to me.

After I entered full-time practice, I remember a troubling question posed by a resident who was on an elective working with me for a month. The resident was a fellow Christian and was also against abortions. As I was about to see a patient who was considering having an IUD, he asked, "Bill, what do you do about IUDs (and the probability that they caused abortion)?" Before he had finished the question, I knew what he was really asking. How could I claim to be pro-life and insert abortifacient devices? I responded somewhat hesitantly, perhaps searching for some firm foundational principle on which to base my thoughts, "You've got to draw the line somewhere. . . I guess it (the conception) is too small. . . . Besides, I'm not really intending to interrupt an already-implanted pregnancy." I remember thinking that I wasn't all that happy with my answers; in fact, my response seemed pretty weak. At the time, I didn't change anything. In retrospect, his question had planted a seed within me.

Years later at a lecture on contraception, I learned of the emerging concerns about IUDs and their potential for serious complications. The speaker thought the potential for harm was so great that he had abandoned inserting them in anyone. While he wasn't opposing IUDs on moral grounds, he provided a strong rationale for me to stop and I immediately did so. I did so under the "cover" of medical concerns for the mother. Nevertheless, looking back, I realize that a nagging burden of my role as a "passive" abortionist had been lifted — at least in part. Still, I would refer for abortions.

Then another small awakening occurred. One morning about ten years ago, I was working in an urgent care facility. A 36-year old narcotic-abusing and alcohol-abusing woman suspected that she was again pregnant. She had previously been pregnant a total of six times. Three of her pregnancies had ended in abortions. The three that she had carried to term had been removed from her care because of her neglect and continuing drug addiction. Her pregnancy test confirmed that she indeed was pregnant for a seventh time and she wanted an abortion. I encouraged her to look at other options. I mentioned support systems and agencies. I offered her free care for the pregnancy (and beyond). These options were rejected. She persisted in her desire to terminate her baby and asked for a referral. Reluctantly, I agreed to help and left the room.

In the hallway, I asked one of the nurses to assist her in "connecting" with an abortion facility. Before I could finish the sentence, the nurse responded, "I don't deal with that." I started another sentence, and, again she interrupted "I'm sorry. I don't deal with that at all." Her response took me aback, yet I respected her stance. In fact, I agreed with it. As she walked away, I stood there in silence. I wondered why I was involving myself in what I thought was wrong.

I decided to change. I re-entered the room and gently re-stated my willingness to help my patient in any and all ways possible, but this time firmly stated that I was unable to help her obtain an abortion. The nurse's courage in living her beliefs had served as a model in helping me to be more consistent myself. Again, in retrospect, I felt a sense of relief. I had rejected my propensity to compromise my own principles.

Still, my practice continued to include other contraceptives as well as sterilization procedures. In fact, I was one of the first physicians in our university practice to learn to insert progestin implants. If there were problems with these choices, I didn't let the conflict rise to a conscious level. On a personal level, my wife and I were increasingly aware of problems with birth control pills and had stopped using contraceptives in our own marriage. We also had joined a more orthodox Catholic parish where the norm among most couples with children was to avoid the use of contraceptives. At the same time, I continued to dispense contraceptives in my practice.

Then about five years ago an epiphany occurred. Marlene and I attended a three-day conference being sponsored by Human Life International held in our own parish hall. The entire conference was devoted to an in-depth look at *Humanae Vitae*, the encyclical written by Pope Paul VI more than two decades earlier. Experts from around the country explained the theological, philosophical, and medical concerns related to all forms of artificial birth control as well as with birth control pills in specific. Within the first half-day of the conference, I understood the need to change. Birth control pills clearly induced a "chemical" abortion in some conceptions. I could not clearly practice in a way that ignored this reality. Furthermore, I came to understand that the whole practice of artificial birth control was against God's plan for married couples.

I knew that I had a decision to make. Having been given these new insights, I knew if I went on prescribing pills, I would be inconsistent at the least and a hypocrite at worst. Alternatively, I could divest myself of any involvement in artificial contraceptives. But was this really a viable alternative? After all, I taught residents and medical students. What would they think? Dispensing contraceptives and family planning procedures such as performing vasectomies had become a big part of my practice. On a personal level, would I be able to continue to teach? What would my colleagues think? I had a large family and I worried about the financial implication of such a decision. I was feeling nervous. I wrestled over the next two and one-half days of the conference. I was afraid to discuss my decision with Marlene, fearing that even a discussion of the issue might limit my options. I might be pressured to embrace a new way of practicing that I wouldn't be able to maintain or that I wouldn't be able to sustain us as a family.

Despite my fear and reluctance to even discuss the issue, I finally made a silent decision and commitment to myself. I would stop using the hormonal contraceptives that I recognized were abortifacient. What's more, I made the commitment to myself to not engage in any medical practice that was in conflict with the clear and consistent teachings of the Roman Catholic Church. This meant I would stop performing vasectomies, assisting with tubal ligation, and would even refrain from referring for any of these procedures. I had come to the recognition that I could not morally help another to do that which is inconsistent with God's plan for married couples. I was still nervous, but I was going to do my best to keep the resolution.

To my surprise, the first patient who asked me for birth control pills was actually appreciative of my perspective. She didn't want to be taking anything that had even a remote risk of acting as an abortifacient. Furthermore, she was excited about the concept of natural family planning and thought her husband would be too. I eagerly responded to her interest and supplied her with information, community resources, and a follow-up appointment. Maybe the new approach wouldn't be as difficult as I thought.

Not so. Over the subsequent month, not all of my patients were as responsive. Some were frankly annoyed. In these cases, after recognizing their frustration, I would ask for their understanding and apologize for the error that they had been scheduled with me for the appointment. I would tell them there would be no charge for the visit. At the same time, having fully explained my personal and religious convictions, I gently but firmly told them I could not help them.

To this day, I've not yet encountered a patient who did not respect my position (just as I respect their option not to conform to my beliefs). While I have lost a few patients, I have gained many more who seek me out because of the change in my practice. Despite my fears about the financial situation, the income that year (and subsequently) has actually been higher than it had been when I was dispensing artificial birth control! For me personally, a weight that I hadn't even recognized has been completely lifted. I think that I am more effective and certainly more consistent with my patients. I believe many couples in my practice have stronger marriages.

As an academic physician, I've even taken the risk of teaching natural family planning (NFP) to residents and students. The title of my talk to them is "Natural Family Planning — The Forgotten Family Planning Option." In general, residents, students and even fellow faculty are astonished to learn that family planning and the spacing of children can be done as reliably with natural means as with hormones— without any side effects!

In summary, my journey toward a fully pro-life position and medical practice has been long and a bit bumpy at times, yet I've never looked back. As I reflect on the roads traveled, I clearly see God's fingerprints at each junction. Once it was a resident's provocative question. Another time it was a colleague or a nurse who modeled a different way to practice. Finally, it was the profound witness for the Truth expressed in *Humanae Vitae*. At each branch in the road, one of God's laborers helped me to be more consistent in applying my faith to my practice. As a result, I now strive to share my new and life-giving paradigm with all who will listen. I think I have become a brighter light to my patients and I'm grateful to each of the guides who He sent to help point the way for me.

Appendix I

Reconsidering *Humanae Vitae*

Father Charles M. Mangan

Humanae Vitae, the papal encyclical authored by Pope Paul VI offers Catholic husbands and wives a meditation on the mystery of life and love. The 30th anniversary of its promulgation on July 25, 1968, gives Catholic couples an excellent opportunity to reconsider its teaching, a teaching that has been reconfirmed dozens of times by Pope John Paul II.

Following are only a few of the points made by Pope Paul in *Humanae Vitae* that can help contemporary Catholic spouses better understand marriage and family:

1. The magisterium, or teaching authority of the Church, has every right to speak about procreation. Why? Because Jesus Christ bestowed upon Peter and the apostles His divine authority to teach His commands and to interpret their meaning and application. This special authority extends not only to Sacred Scripture and the apostolic tradition but also to the Natural Law, which Saint Paul stated might be known by everyone regardless of creed.

2. Husbands and wives are to share everything with each other; nothing is to be withheld. The love between spouses is faithful and exclusive until death. The "responsible exercise of parenthood" demands, in the words of Pope Paul, "that husband and wife recognize fully their own duties toward God, toward themselves, toward

the family, and toward society, in a correct hierarchy of values."

3. The marital act is "noble and worthy" and has two dimensions, the unitive (love-giving) and the procreative (life-giving). The Church has constantly taught that each and every act of marital intercourse "must remain open to the transmission of life." God the Creator has established for all time the inseparable link between unity and procreation in the conjugal act.

4. The "totality" argument that the marital act need not be open each and every time to the possibility of procreation, but that married couples should be receptive at least some of the time during the totality of their marriage to the gift of children, must be rejected. It's immoral to do evil (e.g., using contraception even for a time) so that a supposed good (e.g., conceiving a child when a husband and wife are ready) may result.

5. Direct, procured abortion is intrinsically evil, as are any actions that deliberately make procreation impossible. This includes the use of drugs, such as Depo-Provera and Norplant, which are clearly abortifacient. Many of these chemical abortions parade as contraceptives, but actually prevent implantation of a conceived child.

6. Direct sterilization is intrinsically evil. To cure a disease, however, it's permissible for a man or a woman to undergo a medical treatment that will result in sterility, as long as the sterility isn't directly intended.

7. For "serious" motives, couples may have marital intercourse during the woman's monthly infertile period even though procreation may not result since there are "natural rhythms immanent in the generative functions." The Church teaches that a vast difference exists between contraception and Natural Family Planning (NFP). The former advocates unlimited sexual intimacy between spouses, while the latter makes use of the infertile period only when serious reasons warrant.

Catholic couples may be assured that the Church doesn't shirk her sacred duty to give direction and counsel to them about their grave responsibility to bring forth new life into the world.

While one Christian denomination after another has granted "permission" for their members to use contraception, the Catholic Church stands virtually alone as the major force which refuses to countenance contraception. This fact in itself speaks loudly about the Church's insistence on obeying the law of God, no matter the scorn and outcry received.

Three decades after *Humanae Vitae*, the truth about the gift of children has not changed. Married couples are summoned by the Creator Himself to cooperate in the conception and birth of His sons and daughters.

Pope Paul VI was right. The Church is right. To do the just and moral thing may be difficult, but God won't fail to reward those married couples who have, with His grace, hurdled the obstacles against procreation and generously accepted the treasure of human life.

This article originally appeared in the July 19-25, 1998, issue of "Catholic Faith and Family."

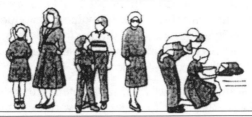

Drs. Hartman, Larimore & Shupe
Family Physicians

June 9, 1995

Dear Patient,

I am writing you to let you know of an important decision that I have made recently. I know that for some of you, this will come as a surprise while others will see this as natural as the bloom that comes from a bud.

The decision I speak of is my desire to no longer prescribe any method of artificial birth control. In concrete terms, this encompasses most forms of contraception, such as birth control pills, vasectomy, tubal ligation the diaphragm, condoms, foam and the other more problematic methods (the IUD, Depo-Provera, Norplant and abortion). Not included in this list is NATURAL FAMILY PLANNING, a totally safe and reliable method of birth control (efficiency rate = 98%). This method also has the advantage of emphasizing mutual responsibility, promoting respect and fostering spouse-to-spouse communication.

The major thrust behind this decision is my desire to be totally Pro-Life in my recommendations. Recently I have come to a greater realization that my role as physician and healer makes certain demands of me. One of these is that I promote those actions which foster respect for the mystery of life, from conception and birth to procreation and the making of new life and finally to death and its entry into the life of the hereafter. Another is that I avoid endorsing those things that result in short term benefits at the expense of your long term health and development: physical, mental, emotional and spiritual. I understand now that the artificial methods of birth control do not fully allow for these benefits.

This decision of mine which I announce to you today has first been discussed with my partners. After thoughtful dialogue and discussion of the ramifications of such a move, they both have given me their full support and encouragement while retaining their right to offer some of the birth control options.

I realize that some of you will be disappointed in this decision. However, I felt a keen obligation to make you aware to this change in my practice, since it may prompt some action or reconsideration on your part.

I would like to assure you that I will continue to provide full service family practice, in particular maternity care and gynecologic issues such as Pap smears, conception counseling and treatment of disease, including menstrual irregularities, ovarian cysts, and infectious diseases, just as I have done in the past. In addition, I consider it one of my most important roles to serve as one who counsels on a broad range of health issues and who encourages you to reach out and fulfill your destiny.

As always, please feel free when you visit to bring up any concerns you have regarding this recent decision. If you find you need some clarification before you visit, you may wish to speak with one of our nurses: Melony, Judy, Leticia or Rosemary. Your health care needs are of paramount importance to us. We strive to assist you when you need help.

In closing, I wish to say that I am honored when you entrust to me your most precious gift: the gift of life and I am grateful for your confidence in me. I pray that I may always be worthy to be of service to you.

With deepest respect,

John R. Hartman, M.D.

APPENDIX III

Why I do not prescribe contraceptives
by Doctor Mark Povich, DO

Several years ago I was presented with information regarding the mechanisms of action of certain contraceptive agents. As one who believes that human life begins at the moment of conception, I was disturbed by portions of the following facts:

A. Oral contraceptives (the "Pill") are believed to have three mechanisms of action:
      1. Prevent ovulation (release of egg by ovary),
      2. Change the cervical mucus to prevent or delay migration of sperm, and
      3. Prevent implantation of an approximately one week old fertilized egg onto the lining of the womb.

While there is currently no test to determine exact frequencies, the third mechanism is thought possibly to occur in anywhere from two to ten percent of female cycles.

B. Certain progestin medications, such as Depo-Provera and Norplant, are similar to the oral contraceptives in mechanism of action, but less effective at preventing ovulation. It is estimated that ovulation occurs in 40-60% of cycles while on these medications. The potential for eggs to be fertilized and then not be allowed to implant increases under these conditions.

C. IUD's (intrauterine devices) have no known effect of preventing ovulation, but work primarily to prevent implantation of the developing embryo (early fertilized egg).

Faced with this knowledge, I could not continue to prescribe medications or devices that I knew had the potential for destroying a life in its early stages. If parents have a child die, they obviously grieve the loss. When there is a stillbirth, parents still grieve even though they never had a chance to see the child living. I have seen many women grieve over a miscarriage in their first two to three months of pregnancy, though they never felt the baby move or even looked pregnant. Nevertheless, each knew the potential of what had been growing in her womb. What about a fertilized egg that has

141

every potential to be a loved child but was never allowed to
implant in Mom's womb? There is no grieving, not because
the woman did not value what was lost, but rather she had
no perception of what was lost. Most women have no knowledge that this is occurring. I cannot in good conscience prescribe treatments that I believe are capable of destroying life
at its earliest stages.

To my patients who share a Christian belief system, please allow me to expand on defining life as beginning at the moment
of conception rather than at implantation or some later time.

1. We cannot accept that Jesus Christ is the Son of
    God unless we accept that He did not have a hu-
    man father but rather that the Holy Spirit was
    His father.

2. We cannot accept that the Holy Spirit was His fa-
    ther unless we accept that His human mother
    was a virgin and there was no opportunity for
    conception by a human father.

3. If we accept the above, we must conclude that
    Jesus Christ began His human existence at the
    time of conception — the fertilization of a hu-
    man egg by the Holy Spirit — rather than His
    spirit indwelling some already developing fetus
    (unborn child).

4. If Jesus Christ had human existence since con-
    ception, why should we think that human life
    begins at some later moment in time?

I would be happy to discuss any of these issues with you.
Thank you.

Mark Povich

Appendix IV

Sources for supportive resources mentioned by the authors (and more):

A. National NFP Teacher Training Programs

1. Billings Ovulation Method Association — USA
   Kay Ek, President
   e-mail: NFPStC@cloudnet.com
   316 North 7th Avenue
   St. Cloud, MN 56303-3631
   320-252-2100 or 888-637-63711.

2. Couple to Couple League
   John F. Kippley, President
   4290 Delphi Pike
   Cincinnati, OH 45238
   513-471-2000

3. Family of the Americas Foundation
   Mercedes Wilson, Executive Director
   P.O. Box 1170
   Dunkirk, MD 20754
   301-627-3346

4. Northwest Family Services, Inc.
   Rose Fuller, Executive Director
   4805 NE Glisan Street
   Portland, OR 97213
   503-215-6377

5. Pope Paul VI Institute
   Dr. Thomas Hilgers, MD, Director
   6901 Mercy Road
   Omaha, NE 68106
   402-390-6600

B. Other Physician Support Organizations

1. American Academy of Natural Family Planning (AANFP)
   Joseph Stanford, MD, President (1998-1999)
   University of Utah
   Department of Family and Prevention Medicine
   50 N. Medical Drive
   Salt Lake City, UT 84132
   801-581-7234 x359

2. Catholic Medical Association
   Paul Byrne, MD, President
   850 Elm Grove Road
   Elm Grove, WI 53122
   414-784-3435

3. Diocesan Development Program for NFP,
   Theresa Notare, Associate Director
   National Conference of Catholic Bishops,
   3211 Fourth Street, NE
   Washington, DC
   202-541-3240/3054

4. One More Soul
   Steve Koob, Director
   OMSoul@juno.com
   www.OMSoul.com
   616 Five Oaks Avenue
   Dayton, OH 45406
   800-307-7685
   Source for:
   "Contraception: Why Not?" tape by Professor Janet E. Smith, *Humanae Vitae* — encyclical letter of Pope Paul VI — translated from Latin by Professor Smith, and many other resources.